The Cardiovascular System at a Glance

PHILIP I. AARONSON PhD
Senior Lecturer in Pharmacology
Guy's, King's and St Thomas' School of Medicine, Dentistry and Biomedical Sciences
King's College, London

JEREMY P.T. WARD PhD
Reader in Respiratory Cell Physiology
Guy's, King's and St Thomas' School of Medicine, Dentistry and Biomedical Sciences
King's College, London

CHARLES M. WIENER MD
Associate Professor of Medicine and Physiology
Johns Hopkins School of Medicine
Baltimore, MD, USA

STEVEN P. SCHULMAN MD
Associate Professor of Medicine
Johns Hopkins School of Medicine
Baltimore, MD, USA

JASWINDER S. GILL MA, MD, FRCP
Consultant Cardiologist
Cardiothoracic Centre
St Thomas' Hospital, London

Blackwell Science

© 1999 by
Blackwell Science Ltd
Editorial Offices:
Osney Mead, Oxford OX2 0EL
25 John Street, London WC1N 2BL
23 Ainslie Place, Edinburgh EH3 6AJ
350 Main Street, Malden
    MA 02148 5018, USA
54 University Street, Carlton
    Victoria 3053, Australia
10, rue Casimir Delavigne
    75006 Paris, France

Other Editorial Offices:
Blackwell Wissenschafts-Verlag GmbH
Kurfürstendamm 57
10707 Berlin, Germany

Blackwell Science KK
MG Kodenmacho Building
7–10 Kodenmacho Nihombashi
Chuo-ku, Tokyo 104, Japan

The right of the Authors to be
identified as the Authors of this Work
has been asserted in accordance
with the Copyright, Designs and
Patents Act 1988.

First published 1999

Set by Graphicraft Limited, Hong Kong
Printed and bound in the UK by
MPG Books Ltd, Bodmin, Cornwall

The Blackwell Science logo is a
trade mark of Blackwell Science Ltd,
registered at the United Kingdom
Trade Marks Registry

DISTRIBUTORS

Marston Book Services Ltd
PO Box 269
Abingdon, Oxon OX14 4YN
(*Orders*: Tel: 01235 465500
            Fax: 01235 465555)

USA
Blackwell Science, Inc.
Commerce Place
350 Main Street
Malden, MA 02148 5018
(*Orders*: Tel: 800 759 6102
                781 388 8250
            Fax: 781 388 8255)

Canada
Login Brothers Book Company
324 Saulteaux Crescent
Winnipeg, Manitoba R3J 3T2
(*Orders*: Tel: 204 837-2987)

Australia
Blackwell Science Pty Ltd
54 University Street
Carlton, Victoria 3053
(*Orders*: Tel: 3 9347 0300
            Fax: 3 9347 5001)

A catalogue record for this title
is available from the British Library

ISBN 0–632–04971–5

Library of Congress
Cataloging-in-publication Data

Aaronson, Philip.
    The cardiovascular system at a glance / Philip Aaronson,
Jeremy Ward, Charles M. Wiener, Steven P. Schulman &
Jaswinder S. Gill.
        p.   cm.
    Includes index.
    ISBN 0–632–04971–5
    1. Cardiovascular system—Physiology.
    2. Cardiovascular system—Pathophysiology.
    I. Ward, Jeremy.   II. Title.
    [DNLM: 1. Cardiovascular System.
WG 100 A113c 1999]
QP 101. A18   1999
616. 1—dc21
DNLM/DLC
for Library of Congress   98–54927
                                                     CIP

For further information on
Blackwell Science, visit our website:
www.blackwell-science.com

Contents

Preface

This book aims to provide a comprehensive yet concise description of the cardiovascular system which integrates normal structure, function and regulation with pathophysiology, pharmacology, and therapeutics. It is directed mainly at preclinical medical students taking systems-based courses. It should, however, serve equally well as an introduction to this subject suitable for other biomedical students and scientists, as well as a focused 'refresher course' for clinicians, nurses and other health care professionals.

The book is divided into 55 chapters, the last four of which are case studies. Each chapter is based around one or two diagrams or tables, and is designed to contain an amount of information roughly equivalent to that typically presented in an hour-long lecture. In addition to incorporating the mainstream topics appropriate for a complete systems-based preclinical medical course on the cardiovascular system, we have also included subjects less commonly encountered by preclinical students. These include chapters on the aetiology of primary hypertension, risk factors for cardiovascular disease, cardiac transplantation, congenital cardiac disease, and mitral and aortic valve disease.

Acknowledgements

We are grateful to the students and fellow academics who read many of the chapters, and offered both criticism and encouragement. We received invaluable advice from Dr Jane Ward, Dr Fred Imms, Dr Richard Leach, Professor Lucilla Poston, Nick Maycock, Aman Bhandari, Vaneeta Sood and, in particular, from Zoë Wardley. We are also grateful to Dr Michael Stein and Charlie Hamlyn, our editors, who put up gracefully with endless missed deadlines and modifications.

Recommended reading

E. Braunwald, ed. *Heart Disease, A Texbook of Cardiovascular Medicine*, 5th edn. WB Saunders, Philadelphia, 1997.

D. Jordan & J. Marshall, eds. *Cardiovascular Regulation*. Portland Press, London, 1995.

J.R. Levick. *An Introduction to Cardiovascular Physiology*, 2nd edn. Butterworth-Heinemann, Oxford, 1995.

L.S. Lilly, ed. *Pathophysiology of Heart Disease*. Lea & Febiger, Philadelphia, 1993.

Sources of illustrations

1 Overview of the cardiovascular system

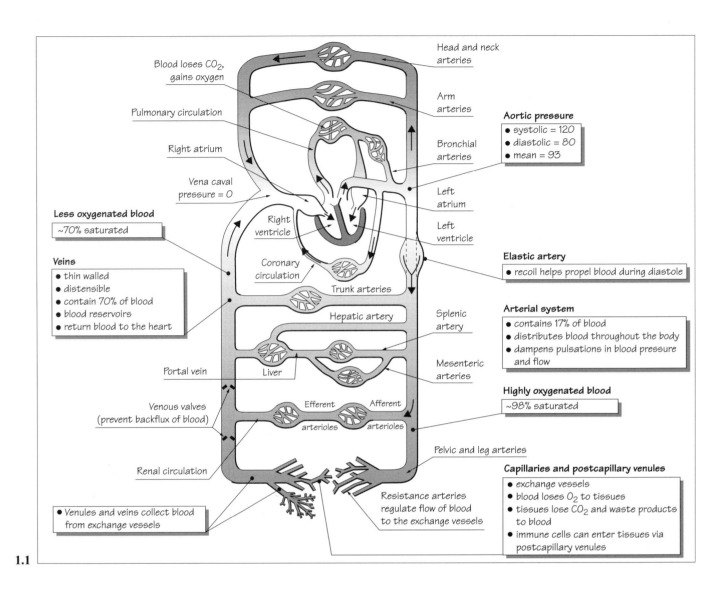

The cardiovascular system is composed of the heart, blood vessels and blood. In simple terms, its main functions are:

1 Distribution of O_2 and nutrients (e.g. glucose, amino acids) to all body tissues.

2 Transportation of CO_2 and metabolic waste products (e.g. urea) from the tissues to the lungs and excretory organs.

3 Distribution of water, electrolytes and hormones throughout the body.

4 Contributing to the infrastructure of the immune system.

5 Thermoregulation.

Blood is composed of **plasma**, an aqueous solution containing electrolytes, proteins and other molecules, in which **cells** are suspended. The cells comprise 40–45% of blood volume and are mainly **erythrocytes**, but also **white blood cells**

and **platelets**. Blood volume is about 5.5 litres in an 'average' 70-kg man.

The figure illustrates the 'plumbing' of the cardiovascular system.

Blood is driven through the cardiovascular system by the **heart**, a muscular pump divided into left and right sides. Each side contains two chambers, an **atrium** and a **ventricle**, composed mainly of cardiac muscle cells. The thin-walled atria serve to fill or 'prime' the thick-walled ventricles, which when full constrict forcefully, creating a pressure head that drives the blood out into the body. Blood enters and leaves each chamber of the heart through separate one-way valves, which open and close reciprocally (i.e. one closes before the other opens) to ensure that flow is unidirectional.

Consider the flow of blood starting with its exit from the left ventricle.

When the ventricles contract, the left ventricular internal pressure rises from 0 to 120 mmHg (atmospheric pressure = 0). As the pressure rises, the aortic valve opens and blood is expelled into the **aorta**, the first and largest artery of the **systemic circulation**. This period of ventricular contraction is termed **systole**. The maximal pressure during systole is called the **systolic pressure**, and it serves both to drive blood through the aorta and to distend the aorta, which is quite elastic. The aortic valve then closes, and the left ventricle relaxes so that it can be refilled with blood from the left atrium via the mitral valve. The period of relaxation is called **diastole**. During diastole aortic blood flow and pressure diminish but do not fall to zero, because *elastic recoil* of the aorta continues to exert a **diastolic pressure** on the blood, which gradually falls to a minimum level of about 80 mmHg. The difference between systolic and diastolic pressures is termed the **pulse pressure**. **Mean aortic pressure** is pressure averaged over the entire cardiac cycle. Because the heart spends approximately 60% of the cardiac cycle in diastole, the mean aortic pressure is approximately equal to the diastolic pressure + one-third of the pulse pressure, rather than to the arithmetic average of the systolic and diastolic pressures.

The blood flows from the aorta into the **major arteries**, each of which supplies blood to an organ or body region. These arteries divide and subdivide into smaller **muscular arteries**, which eventually give rise to the **arterioles**—arteries with diameters of < 100 μm. Blood enters the arterioles at a mean pressure of about 60–70 mmHg.

The walls of the arteries and arterioles have circumferentially arranged layers of **smooth muscle cells**. The lumen of the entire vascular system is lined by a monolayer of **endothelial cells**. These cells secrete vasoactive substances and serve as a barrier, restricting and controlling the movement of fluid, molecules and cells into and out of the vasculature.

The arterioles lead to the smallest vessels, the **capillaries**, which form a dense network within all body tissues. The capillary wall is a layer of overlapping endothelial cells, with no smooth muscle cells. The pressure in the capillaries ranges from about 25 mmHg on the arterial side to 15 mmHg at the venous end. The capillaries converge into small **venules**, which also have thin walls of mainly endothelial cells. The venules merge into larger venules, with an increasing content of smooth muscle cells as they widen. These then converge to become **veins**, which progressively join to give rise to the **superior** and **inferior venae cavae**, through which blood returns to the right side of the heart. Veins have a larger diameter than arteries, and thus offer relatively little resistance to flow. The small pressure gradient between venules (15 mmHg) and the venae cavae (0 mmHg) is therefore sufficient to drive blood back to the heart.

Blood from the venae cavae enters the **right atrium**, and then the **right ventricle** through the **tricuspid valve**. Contraction of the right ventricle, simultaneous with that of the left ventricle, forces blood through the pulmonary valve into the pulmonary artery, which progressively subdivides to form the arteries, arterioles and capillaries of the **pulmonary circulation**. The pulmonary circulation is shorter and has a much lower pressure than the systemic circulation, with systolic and diastolic pressures of about 25 and 10 mmHg, respectively. The pulmonary capillary network within the lungs surrounds the alveoli of the lungs, allowing exchange of CO_2 for O_2. Oxygenated blood enters pulmonary venules and veins, and then the **left atrium**, which pumps it into the left ventricle for the next systemic cycle.

The output of the right ventricle is slightly lower than that of the left ventricle. This is because 1–2% of the systemic blood flow never reaches the right atrium, but is shunted to the left side of the heart via the bronchial circulation (Fig. 1.1) and the small fraction of coronary blood flow which drains into the thebesian veins (see Chapter 24).

Blood vessel functions

Each vessel type has important functions in addition to being a conduit for blood.

The branching system of elastic and muscular arteries progressively reduces the pulsations in blood pressure and flow imposed by the intermittent ventricular contractions.

The smallest arteries and arterioles play a crucial role in regulating the amount of blood flowing to the tissues by dilating or constricting. This function is regulated by the sympathetic nervous system, and factors generated locally in tissues. These vessels are referred to as **resistance arteries**, because their constriction resists the flow of blood.

Capillaries and small venules are the **exchange vessels**. Through their walls, gases, fluids and molecules are transferred between blood and tissues. White blood cells can also pass through the venule walls to fight infection in the tissues.

Venules can constrict to offer resistance to the bloodflow, and the ratio of arteriolar and venular resistance exerts an important influence on the movement of fluid between capillaries and tissues, thereby affecting blood volume.

The veins are thin walled and very *distensible*, and therefore contain about 70% of all blood in the cardiovascular system. The arteries contain just 17% of total blood volume. Veins and venules thus serve as volume reservoirs, which can shift blood from the peripheral circulation into the heart and arteries by constricting. In doing so, they are able to increase the **cardiac output** (volume of blood pumped by the heart per unit time), and they are also able to maintain the blood pressure and tissue perfusion in essential organs if **haemorrhage** (blood loss) occurs.

2 Gross anatomy and histology of the heart

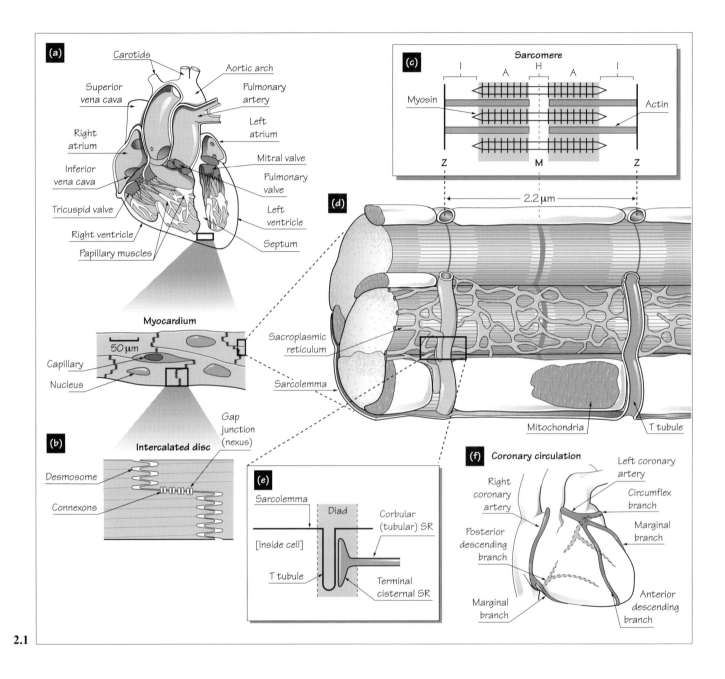

2.1

Gross anatomy of the heart (Fig. 2.1a)

The heart consists of four chambers. Blood flows into the right atrium via the superior and inferior venae cavae. The left and right atria connect to the ventricles via the mitral (two cusps) and tricuspid (three cusps) atrioventricular (AV) valves, respectively. The AV valves are passive and close when the ventricular pressure exceeds that in the atrium. They are prevented from being everted into the atria during systole by fine cords (**chordae tendineae**) attached between the free margins of the

cusps and the papillary muscles, which contract during systole. The outflow from the right ventricle passes through the pulmonary semilunar valve to the pulmonary artery, and that from the left ventricle enters the aorta via the aortic semilunar valve. These valves close passively at the end of systole, when ventricular pressure falls below that of the arteries. Both semilunar valves have three cusps.

The cusps or leaflets of the cardiac valves are formed of fibrous connective tissue, covered in a thin layer of cells similar to and contiguous with the **endocardium** (AV valves and ventricular surface of semilunar valves) and **endothelium** (vascular side of semilunar valves). When closed, the cusps form a tight seal (come to apposition) at the **commissures** (line at which the edges of the leaflets meet).

The atria and ventricles are separated by a band of fibrous connective tissue called the **annulus fibrosus**, which provides a skeleton for attachment of the muscle and insertion of the valves. It also prevents electrical conduction between the atria and ventricles except at the **atrioventricular node** (AVN). This is situated near the interatrial septum and the mouth of the coronary sinus and is an important element of the cardiac electrical conduction system.

The ventricles fill during diastole; at the initiation of the heart beat the atria contract and complete ventricular filling. As the ventricles contract the pressure rises sharply, closing the AV valves. When ventricular pressure exceeds the pulmonary artery or aortic pressure, the semilunar valves open and ejection occurs (see Chapter 13). As systole ends and ventricular pressure falls, the semilunar valves are closed by backflow of blood from the arteries.

The force of contraction is generated by the muscle of the heart, the **myocardium**. The atrial walls are thin. The greater pressure generated by the left ventricle compared with the right is reflected by its greater wall thickness. The inside of the heart is covered in a thin layer of cells called the **endocardium**, which is similar to the endothelium of blood vessels. The outer surface of the myocardium is covered by the **epicardium**, a layer of mesothelial cells. The whole heart is enclosed in the **pericardium**, a thin fibrous sheath or sac, which prevents excessive enlargement. The **pericardial space** contains interstitial fluid as a lubricant.

Structure of the myocardium

The myocardium consists of **cardiac myocytes** (*muscle cells*) that show a striated subcellular structure, although they are less organized than skeletal muscle. The cells are relatively small ($100 \times 20 \ \mu m$) and branched, with a single nucleus, and are rich in mitochondria. They are connected together as a network by **intercalated discs** (Fig. 2.1b), where the cell membranes are closely opposed. The intercalated discs provide both a structural attachment by 'glueing' the cells together at **desmosomes**, and an electrical connection through **gap junctions** formed of pores made up of proteins called **connexons**. As a result, the myocardium acts as a **functional syncytium**, in other words as a single functional unit, even though the individual cells are still separate. The gap junctions play a vital role in conduction of the electrical impulse through the myocardium (see Chapter 15).

The myocytes contain **actin** and **myosin** filaments which form the contractile apparatus, and exhibit the classical M and Z lines and A, H and I bands (Fig. 2.1c). The intercalated discs always coincide with a Z line, as it is here that the actin filaments are anchored to the cytoskeleton. At the Z lines the **sarcolemma** (cell membrane) forms tubular invaginations into the cells known as the **transverse (T) tubular system**. The **sarcoplasmic reticulum** (SR) is less extensive than in skeletal muscle, and runs generally in parallel with the length of the cell (Fig. 2.1d). Close to the T tubules the SR forms **terminal cisternae** that with the T tubule make up **diads** (Fig. 2.1e), an important component of excitation-contraction coupling (see Chapter 11). The typical *triad* seen in skeletal muscle is less often present. The T tubules and SR never physically join, but are separated by a narrow gap. The myocardium has an extensive system of capillaries.

Coronary circulation (Fig. 2.1f)

The heart has a rich blood supply, derived from the **left and right coronary arteries**. These arise separately from the aortic sinus at the base of the aorta, behind the cusps of the aortic valve. They are not blocked by the cusps during systole because of eddy currents, and remain patent throughout the cardiac cycle. The **right coronary artery** runs forward between the pulmonary trunk and right atrium, to the AV sulcus. As it descends to the lower margin of the heart, it divides to **posterior descending** and **right marginal** branches. The **left coronary artery** runs behind the pulmonary trunk and forward between it and the left atrium. It divides into the **circumflex**, **left marginal** and **anterior descending** branches. There are anastomoses between the left and right marginal branches, and the anterior and posterior descending arteries, although these are not sufficient to maintain perfusion if one side of the coronary circulation is occluded.

Most of the blood returns to the right atrium via the **coronary sinus**, and **anterior cardiac veins**. The **large** and **small** coronary veins run parallel to the left and right coronary arteries, respectively, and empty into the sinus. Numerous other small vessels empty into the cardiac chambers directly, including **thebesian veins** and **arteriosinusoidal vessels**.

The coronary circulation is capable of developing a good collateral system in ischaemic heart disease, when a branch or branches are occluded by, for example, atheromatous plaques. Most of the left ventricle is supplied by the left coronary artery, and occlusion can therefore be very dangerous. The AVN and **sinus node** are supplied by the right coronary artery in the majority of people; disease in this artery can cause a slow heart rate and AV block (see Chapters 10, 15).

3 Vascular anatomy

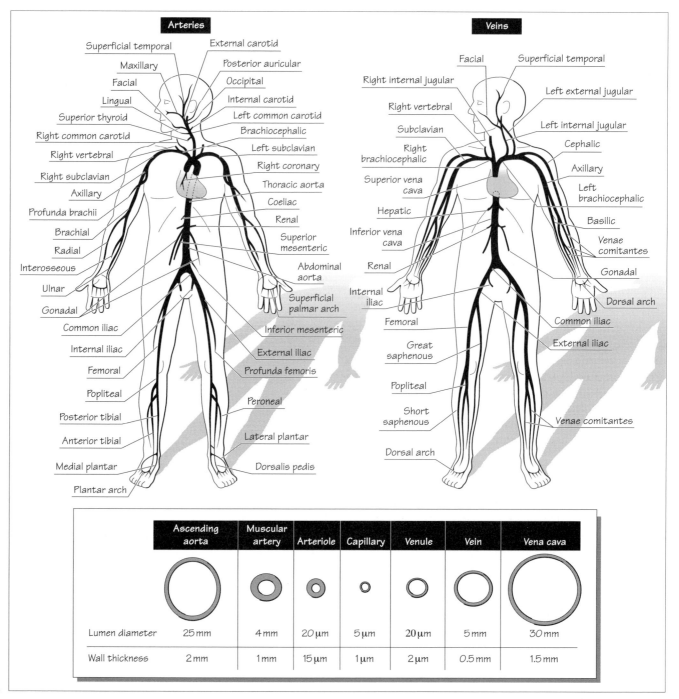

	Ascending aorta	Muscular artery	Arteriole	Capillary	Venule	Vein	Vena cava
Lumen diameter	25 mm	4 mm	20 μm	5 μm	20 μm	5 mm	30 mm
Wall thickness	2 mm	1 mm	15 μm	1 μm	2 μm	0.5 mm	1.5 mm

3.1

The blood vessels of the cardiovascular system are for convenience of description classified into **arteries** (elastic and muscular), **resistance vessels** (small arteries and arterioles), **capillaries**, **venules** and **veins**. Typical dimensions for the different types of vessel are illustrated.

The systemic circulation

Arteries

The **systemic (or greater) circulation** begins with the pumping of blood by the left ventricle into the largest artery, the **aorta**. This ascends from the top of the heart, bends downward at the *aortic arch* and descends just anterior to the spinal column. The aorta bifurcates into the left and right *iliac arteries*, which supply the pelvis and legs. The major arteries supplying the head, the arms and the heart arise from the aortic arch, and the main arteries supplying the visceral organs branch from the descending aorta. All of the major organs except the liver (see below) are therefore supplied with blood by arteries which arise from the aorta. The fundamentally *parallel* organization of the systemic vasculature has a number of advantages over the alternative *series* arrangement, in which blood would flow sequentially through one organ after another. The parallel arrangement of the vascular system ensures that the supply of blood to each organ is relatively independent, is driven by a large pressure head, and also that each organ receives highly oxygenated blood.

The aorta and its major branches (***brachiocephalic***, ***common carotid***, ***subclavian*** and ***common iliac*** arteries) are termed **elastic arteries**. In addition to conducting blood away from the heart, these arteries distend during systole and recoil during diastole, damping the pulse wave and evening out the discontinuous flow of blood created by the heart's intermittent pumping action.

Elastic arteries branch to give rise to **muscular arteries** with relatively thicker walls; this prevents their collapse when joints bend. The muscular arteries give rise to **resistance vessels**, so named because they present the greatest part of the resistance of the vasculature to the flow of blood. These are sometimes subclassified into *small arteries*, which have multiple layers of smooth muscle cells in their walls, and *arterioles*, which have one or two layers of smooth muscle cells. Resistance vessels have the highest wall/lumen ratio in the vasculature. The degree of constriction or **tone** of these vessels regulates the amount of blood flowing to each small area of tissue. All but the smallest resistance vessels tend to be heavily innervated (especially in the *splanchnic*, *renal* and *cutaneous* vasculatures) by the **sympathetic nervous system**, the activity of which usually causes them to constrict (see Chapter 27).

Arterial anastomoses

In addition to branching to give rise to smaller vessels, arteries and arterioles may also merge to form ***anastomoses***. These are found in many circulations (e.g. the brain, mesentery, uterus, around joints) and provide an alternative supply of blood if one artery is blocked. If this occurs, the anastamosing artery gradually enlarges, providing a **collateral circulation**.

The smallest arterioles, capillaries and postcapillary venules comprise the **microcirculation**; the structure and function of which is described in Chapters 19 and 20.

Veins

The venous system can be divided into the **venules**, which contain one or two layers of smooth muscle cells, and the **veins**. The veins of the limbs, particularly the legs, contain paired semilunar **valves** which ensure that the blood cannot move backwards. These are orientated so that they are pressed against the venous wall when the blood is flowing forward, but are forced out to occlude the lumen when the blood flow reverses.

The veins from the head, neck and arms come together to form the ***superior vena cava***, and those from the lower part of the body merge into the ***inferior vena cava***. These deliver blood to the right atrium, which pumps it into the right ventricle.

The one or two veins draining a body region typically run next to the artery supplying that region. This promotes heat conservation, because at low temperatures the warmer arterial blood gives up its heat to the cooler venous blood, rather than to the external environment. The pulsations of the artery caused by the heart beat also aid the venous flow of blood.

The pulmonary circulation

The **pulmonary (or lesser) circulation** begins when blood is pumped by the right ventricle into the ***main pulmonary artery***, which immediately bifurcates into the ***right*** and ***left pulmonary arteries*** supplying each lung. This 'venous' blood is oxygenated during its passage through the pulmonary capillaries. It then returns to the heart via the ***pulmonary veins*** to the left atrium, which pumps it into the left ventricle. The metabolic demands of the lungs are not met by the pulmonary circulation, but by the **bronchial circulation**. This arises from the ***intercostal arteries***, which branch from the aorta. Most of the veins of the bronchial circulation terminate in the right atrium, but some drain into the pulmonary veins (see Chapter 25).

The splanchnic circulation

The arrangement of the **splanchnic circulation** (liver and digestive organs) is a partial exception to the parallel organization of the systemic vasculature (see Fig. 1.1). Although a fraction of the blood supply to the liver is provided by the hepatic artery, the liver receives most (~70%) of its blood via the ***portal vein***. This vessel carries venous blood that has passed through the capillary beds of the stomach, spleen, pancreas and intestine. Most of the liver's circulation is therefore *in series* with that of the digestive organs. This arrangement facilitates hepatic uptake of nutrients and detoxification of foreign substances which have been absorbed during digestion. This type of sequential perfusion of two capillary beds is referred to as a **portal circulation**. A somewhat different type of portal circulation is also found within the kidney.

The lymphatic system

The body contains a parallel circulatory system of **lymphatic vessels** and **nodes** (see Chapter 20). The lymphatic system functions to return to the cardiovascular system the approximately 8 L/day of interstitial fluid that leaves the exchange vessels to enter body tissues. The larger lymphatic vessels pass through nodes containing lymphocytes, which act to mount an immune response to microbes, bacterial toxins and other foreign material carried into the lymphatic system with the interstitial fluid.

4 Vascular histology and smooth muscle cell ultrastructure

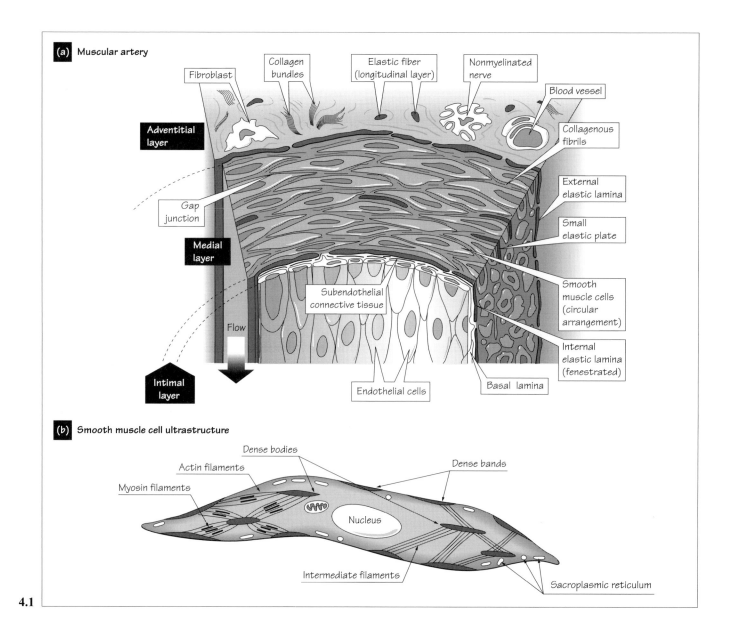

(a) Muscular artery

- Fibroblast
- Collagen bundles
- Elastic fiber (longitudinal layer)
- Nonmyelinated nerve
- Blood vessel
- Collagenous fibrils
- Adventitial layer
- Gap junction
- External elastic lamina
- Small elastic plate
- Medial layer
- Subendothelial connective tissue
- Smooth muscle cells (circular arrangement)
- Internal elastic lamina (fenestrated)
- Flow
- Intimal layer
- Endothelial cells
- Basal lamina

(b) Smooth muscle cell ultrastructure

- Dense bodies
- Actin filaments
- Dense bands
- Myosin filaments
- Nucleus
- Intermediate filaments
- Sacroplasmic reticulum

4.1

Larger blood vessels share a common three-layered structure. Figure 4.1(a) illustrates the arrangement of these layers, or *tunics*, in a muscular artery.

A thin inner layer, the **tunica intima**, comprises an *endothelial cell* monolayer (*endothelium*) supported by connective tissue. The endothelial cells lining the vascular lumen are sealed to each other by *tight junctions*, which restrict the diffusion of large molecules across the endothelium. The endothelial cells play a crucial role in controlling vascular permeability, vasoconstriction, angiogenesis (growth of new blood vessels) and regulation of coagulation. The intima is relatively thicker in larger arteries, and contains some smooth muscle cells in large and medium sized arteries and veins.

The thick middle layer, the **tunica media**, is separated from the intima by a fenestrated (perforated) sheath, the *internal elastic lamina*, mostly composed of elastin. The media contains *smooth muscle cells* embedded in an extracellular matrix composed mainly of collagen, elastin and proteoglycans. The cells are shaped like elongated and irregular spindles or cylinders with tapering ends, and are 15–100 μm long. In the arterial system, they are orientated circularly or in a low-pitch spiral, so that the vascular lumen is narrowed when they contract. Individual cells are long enough to wrap around small arterioles several times.

Adjacent smooth muscle cells form **gap junctions**. These are areas of close cellular contact in which arrays of large channels called **connexons** span both cell membranes, allowing ions to flow from one cell to the other. The smooth muscle cells therefore form a **syncitium**, in which depolarization spreads from each cell to its neighbours.

An *external elastic lamina* separates the tunica media from the outer layer, the **tunica adventitia**. This contains collagenous tissue supporting *fibroblasts* and *nerves*. In large arteries and veins, the adventitia contains **vasa vasorum**, small blood vessels which also penetrate into the outer portion of the media and supply the vascular wall with oxygen and nutrients.

Although arteries and veins share the basic three-layered structure, the layers are less distinct in the venous system. Compared to arteries, veins have a thinner tunica media containing a smaller amount of smooth muscle cells, which also tend to have a more random orientation.

The protein **elastin** is found mainly in the arteries. Molecules of elastin are arranged into a network of randomly coiled fibres. These molecular 'springs' allow arteries to expand during systole and then rebound during diastole to keep the blood flowing forward. This is particularly important in the aorta and other large elastic arteries, in which the media contains fenestrated sheets of elastin separating the smooth muscle cells into multiple concentric layers (**lamellae**).

The fibrous protein **collagen** is present in all three layers of the vascular wall, and functions as a framework that anchors the smooth muscle cells in place. At high internal pressures, the collagen network becomes very rigid, limiting vascular distensibility. This is particularly important in veins, which have a higher collagen content than arteries.

Exchange vessel structure

Capillaries and postcapillary venules are tubes formed of a single layer of overlapping endothelial cells. This is supported and surrounded on the external side by the *basal lamina*, a 50–100 nm-thick layer of fibrous proteins including collagen, and glycoproteins. *Pericytes*, isolated cells which can give rise to smooth muscle cells during angiogenesis, adhere to the outside of the basal lamina, especially in postcapillary venules. The lumenal side of the endothelium is coated by *glycocalyx*, a dense glycoprotein network attached to the cell membrane.

There are three types of capillaries, and these differ in their locations and permeabilities. Their structures are illustrated in Chapter 19.

Continuous capillaries occur in skin, muscles, lungs and the central nervous system. They have a low permeability to molecules that cannot pass readily through cell membranes, owing to the presence of tight junctions which bring the overlapping membranes of adjacent endothelial cells into close contact. The tight junctions run around the perimeter of each cell, forming a seal restricting the paracellular flow of molecules of MW > 10 000. These junctions are especially tight in most capillaries of the central nervous system, and form an integral part of the **blood–brain barrier** (see Chapter 19).

Fenestrated capillaries are much more permeable than continuous capillaries. These are found in endocrine glands, renal glomeruli, intestinal villi and other tissues in which large amounts of fluid or metabolites enter or leave capillaries. In addition to having leakier intercellular junctions, the endothelial cells of these capillaries contain *fenestrae*, circular pores of diameter 50–100 nm spanning areas of the cells where the cytoplasm is thinned. Except in the renal glomeruli, fenestrae are usually covered by a thin perforated diaphragm.

Discontinuous capillaries or **sinusoids** are found in liver, spleen and bone marrow. These are large irregularly shaped capillaries with gaps between the endothelial cells wide enough to allow large proteins and even erythrocytes to cross the capillary wall.

Smooth muscle cell ultrastructure

The cytoplasm of vascular smooth muscle cells contains thin **actin** and thick **myosin** filaments (Fig. 4.1b). Instead of being aligned into sarcomeres as in cardiac myocytes, groups of actin filaments running roughly parallel to the long axis of the cell are anchored at one end into elongated **dense bodies** in the cytoplasm and **dense bands** along the inner face of the cell membrane. Dense bodies and bands are linked by bundles of **intermediate filaments** composed mainly of the proteins **desmin** and **vimentin** to form the **cytoskeleton**, an internal scaffold giving the cell its shape. The free ends of the actin filaments interdigitate with myosin filaments. The myosin crossbridges are structured so that the actin filaments on either side of a myosin filament are pulled in opposite directions during crossbridge cycling (see Chapter 8). This draws the dense bodies towards each other, causing the cytoskeleton, and therefore the cell, to become shorter and fatter. The dense bands are attached to the extracellular matrix by membrane-spanning **integrins**, allowing force development to be distributed through the entire vascular wall.

The **sarcoplasmic reticulum (SR**, also termed smooth endoplasmic reticulum) occupies 2–6% of cell volume. This network of tubes and flattened sacs permeates the cell and contains a high concentration ($\sim$50 mmol/L) of Ca^{2+}. Elements of the SR closely approach the cell membrane. Several types of Ca^{2+}-regulated ion channels and transporters have been found to be concentrated in these areas of the plasmalemma, which may have an important role in cellular excitation.

The nucleus is located in the central part of the cell. Organelles including rough endoplasmic reticulum, Golgi complex and mitochondria are mainly found in the perinuclear region.

5 Constituents of blood

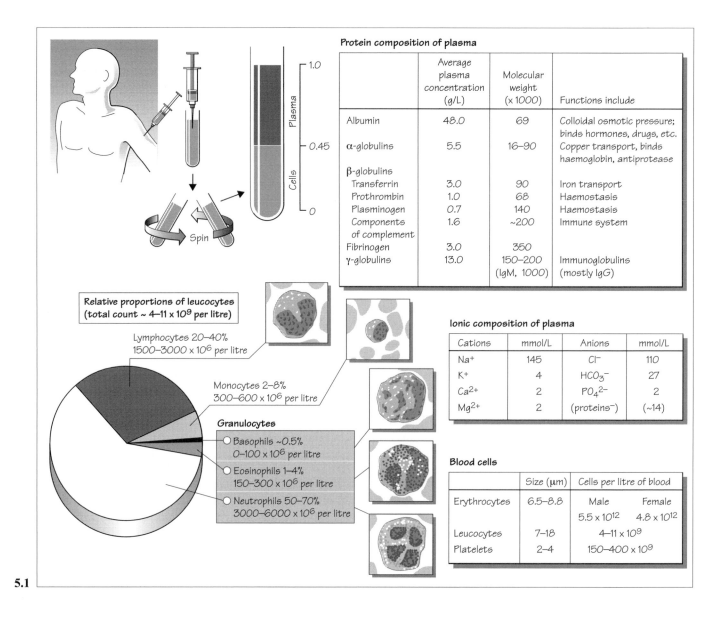

Protein composition of plasma

	Average plasma concentration (g/L)	Molecular weight (x 1000)	Functions include
Albumin	48.0	69	Colloidal osmotic pressure; binds hormones, drugs, etc.
α-globulins	5.5	16–90	Copper transport, binds haemoglobin, antiprotease
β-globulins			
Transferrin	3.0	90	Iron transport
Prothrombin	1.0	68	Haemostasis
Plasminogen	0.7	140	Haemostasis
Components of complement	1.6	~200	Immune system
Fibrinogen	3.0	350	
γ-globulins	13.0	150–200 (IgM, 1000)	Immunoglobulins (mostly IgG)

Relative proportions of leucocytes (total count ~ 4–11 x 10⁹ per litre)

Lymphocytes 20–40%
1500–3000 x 10⁶ per litre

Monocytes 2–8%
300–600 x 10⁶ per litre

Granulocytes

○ Basophils ~0.5%
0–100 x 10⁶ per litre

○ Eosinophils 1–4%
150–300 x 10⁶ per litre

○ Neutrophils 50–70%
3000–6000 x 10⁶ per litre

Ionic composition of plasma

Cations	mmol/L	Anions	mmol/L
Na⁺	145	Cl⁻	110
K⁺	4	HCO₃⁻	27
Ca²⁺	2	PO₄²⁻	2
Mg²⁺	2	(proteins⁻)	(~14)

Blood cells

	Size (μm)	Cells per litre of blood	
		Male	Female
Erythrocytes	6.5–8.8	5.5 x 10¹²	4.8 x 10¹²
Leucocytes	7–18	4–11 x 10⁹	
Platelets	2–4	150–400 x 10⁹	

5.1

The primary function of blood is to deliver O_2 and energy sources to the tissues, and to remove CO_2 and waste products. It contains important elements of the defence and immune systems, is important for the regulation of temperature, and transports hormones and other signalling molecules between tissues. In a 70-kg man blood volume is ~5500 ml, or 8% of body weight. Blood consists of **plasma** and **blood cells**. If 100 ml of blood is spun in a centrifuge, the cells sediment and this **packed cell volume** (PCV, haematocrit) is normally ~45 ml (0.45) in men, less (~0.42) in women.

Plasma

The plasma volume is ~5% of the body weight. It consists of ions in solution and a wide range of plasma proteins. After clotting a straw-coloured fluid called **serum** remains, which differs from plasma only in that fibrinogen and other clotting factors have been removed. The plasma has an **osmolarity** of ~290 mosm/L, mostly due to the dissolved ions and small diffusible molecules (glucose and urea). These diffusible entities exert the **crystalloid osmotic pressure**. Proteins do not pass through capillary walls easily, and are responsible for the **colloidal osmotic pressure** (or **oncotic** pressure) of the plasma. This has a normal value of ~25 mmHg, and is critical for fluid transfer across the capillary wall. Maintenance of plasma osmolarity is vital for the regulation of tissue cell volume and blood volume. Increased crystalloid osmotic pressure stimulates reabsorbtion of water by the kidney, and increases in blood volume. Decreased colloidal osmotic pressure (e.g. low plasma albumin) reduces reabsorbtion of fluid from tissues back into the blood, and leads to **oedema** (see Chapter 20).

Ionic composition

Na^+ is the most prevalent ion in the plasma, and the main determinant of plasma osmolarity and thus blood volume. The concentration of the major ions is shown in the figure, but others are present in smaller amounts (e.g. trace elements). Changes in ionic concentration can have major consequences for excitable tissues (e.g. K^+, Ca^{2+}). Na^+, K^+ and Cl^- are completely dissociated in the plasma, but Ca^{2+} and Mg^{2+} are partly bound to plasma proteins, so that the free concentration is ~50% of the total.

Proteins

Normal total plasma protein concentration is 65–83 g/L; as proteins vary widely in molecular weight the molar concentration is an approximation. Most plasma proteins other than γ-globulins (see below) are synthesized in the liver. Proteins can ionize either as acids or bases because of the presence of both NH_2 and COOH groups. At pH 7.4 they are mostly in the anionic (acidic) form. Their ability to accept or donate H^+ means they can act as buffers, although they account for only ~15% of the buffering capacity of blood. Plasma proteins have an important transport function. They bind with many hormones (e.g. cortisol and thyroxine) and metals (e.g. iron), and are important for blood transport of many drugs, to which they also bind. They may therefore modulate the free concentration of such agents, and thus their biological activity.

Types of plasma protein

Plasma proteins are classified into **albumin** (~48 g/L), **globulin** (~25 g/L) and **fibrinogen** (~2–4 g/L) fractions. Globulins are further classified as α-, β- and γ-globulins, each of which may include many different proteins. β-globulins include transferrin (iron transport), components of complement (immune system), and prothrombin and plasminogen, which with fibrinogen are involved in blood clotting (see Chapter 7). The most important γ-globulins are the immunoglobulins.

Blood cells

In the adult, all blood cells are produced in the **red bone marrow**, although in the fetus, and following bone marrow damage in the adult, they are also produced in the liver and spleen. The marrow contains a small number of **uncommitted stem cells**, which differentiate into specific **committed stem cells** for each blood cell type. The average number of the main types of cell is shown in the figure.

Erythrocytes

Erythrocytes (red cells) are by far the most numerous cells in the blood, with ~5.5 × 10^{12}/L in males (red cell count, RCC).

The haemoglobin they contain is responsible for carriage of O_2, and plays an important role in acid–base buffering. Erythrocytes are biconcave discs and have no nucleus. Their shape and flexibility allows them to deform easily and pass through the capillaries. The erythrocyte sedimentation rate (ESR) is the rate at which cells sediment from blood when allowed to stand in the presence of an anticoagulant. This is increased when cells stack together (form *rouleaux*), and in pregnancy and inflammatory disease. It is decreased by low plasma fibrinogen. Erythrocytes have a normal volume of 85 fl (85 × 10^{-15}/L; mean cell volume, MCV), and ~30 pg of haemoglobin (30 × 10^{-12}/g; mean cell haemoglobin, MCH). The mean cell haemoglobin concentration (MCHC) is thus ~350 g/L. Blood contains ~160 g (male) and ~140 g (female) of haemoglobin per litre. Erythrocytes have an average lifespan of 120 days. Their formation (erythropoiesis), and erythrocyte-related diseases are discussed in Chapter 6.

$$MCV = \frac{PCV}{RCC}; \quad MCH = \frac{Hb}{RCC}; \quad MCHC = \frac{MCH}{MCV} \text{ or } \frac{Hb}{PCV}$$

Leucocytes (white cells)

Leucocytes defend the body against infection by foreign material. The normal total count in adults is 4–11 × 10^9/L, although considerable variations occur. In the newborn the count is ~20 × 10^9/L. Three main types are present in blood: **granulocytes**, **lymphocytes** and **monocytes**. Granulocytes are further classified as **neutrophils**, containing neutral-staining granules, **eosinophils** containing acid-staining granules, and **basophils** containing basic-staining granules. All are involved in the inflammatory response and release inflammatory mediators.

Neutrophils migrate to areas of infection (**chemotaxis**) and destroy bacteria by **phagocytosis**. They have a very short half-life of ~6 h. Eosinophils are less motile than neutrophils and are effective against larger parasites. They are increased in allergic diseases. Basophils contain histamine and heparin and are similar to tissue **mast** cells.

Lymphocytes originate in the marrow but mature in the lymph nodes, thymus and spleen before returning to the circulation. Most remain in the lymphatic system. They are critical components of the **immune** system and produce immunoglobulins (antibodies).

Monocytes have a clear cytoplasm and are larger than granulocytes. After formation in the marrow they circulate in the blood for ~72 h before entering the tissues and becoming **macrophages**, to form the **reticulo-endothelial system** in the liver, spleen and lymph nodes.

Platelets

Platelets are small (~3 μm) vesicle-like structures formed from **megakaryocytes** in the bone marrow. They contain dense granules, microtubules and lyosomes, and have membrane receptors for ADP and collagen. The granules contain serotonin (5-HT) and ADP. They play an important role in **haemostasis** (see Chapter 7). Platelets have a lifespan of ~4 days.

6 Erythropoiesis, haemoglobin and anaemia

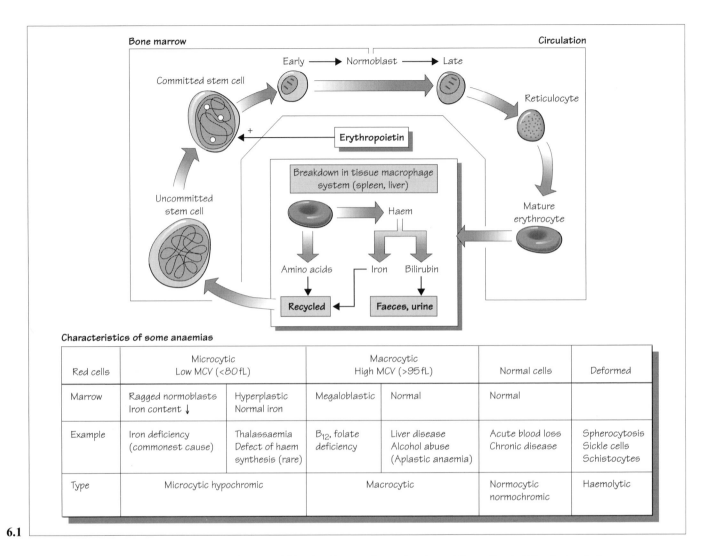

Bone marrow | Circulation

Characteristics of some anaemias

Red cells	Microcytic Low MCV (<80 fL)		Macrocytic High MCV (>95 fL)		Normal cells	Deformed
Marrow	Ragged normoblasts Iron content ↓	Hyperplastic Normal iron	Megaloblastic	Normal	Normal	
Example	Iron deficiency (commonest cause)	Thalassaemia Defect of haem synthesis (rare)	B_{12}, folate deficiency	Liver disease Alcohol abuse (Aplastic anaemia)	Acute blood loss Chronic disease	Spherocytosis Sickle cells Schistocytes
Type	Microcytic hypochromic		Macrocytic		Normocytic normochromic	Haemolytic

6.1

Erythropoiesis leads to the formation of new red blood cells (**erythrocytes**). **Anaemia** is any condition in which there is a reduced blood haemoglobin, resulting in impaired ability of the blood to transport O_2. Some anaemias are associated with abnormal haemoglobins.

Erythropoiesis

Erythrocytes originate from **committed stem cells** in the bone marrow of the adult, and liver and spleen of the fetus. Damage to the marrow can result in erythropoiesis from the liver and spleen of adults. Committed stem cells differentiate into **erythroblasts (early normoblasts)**, which are relatively large (~15 μm) and nucleated. As differentiation proceeds the cells shrink, haemoglobin is synthesized, and in the **late normoblast** the nucleus breaks up and disappears. The young erythrocyte shows a reticulum on staining, and is called a **reticulocyte**. As it ages, the reticulum disappears and the characteristic biconcave

shape develops. Normally 1–2% of circulating red cells are reticulocytes. This increases when erythropoiesis is enhanced, for example by increased **erythropoietin**. About 2×10^{11} erythrocytes are produced from the marrow each day.

Erythropoietin is a glycoprotein hormone produced mainly by the kidneys in adults. In the fetus the main source is the liver. Erythropoietin increases the number of committed stem cells and promotes the production of erythrocytes. The key stimulus for increased erythropoietin is hypoxia. Altitude and chronic respiratory diseases cause the P_{O_2} of the blood to fall, and there is a greatly increased number of erythrocytes (**polycythaemia**) and haematocrit. In kidney disease, chronic inflammation and cirrhosis of the liver erythropoietin levels can fall, resulting in anaemia.

Erythrocytes are destroyed by **macrophages** in the liver and spleen after ~120 days. The spleen also sequesters and eradicates defective erythrocytes. The haem group is split from haemoglobin and converted to **biliverdin** and then **bilirubin**.

The iron is conserved and recycled via **transferrin**, an iron transport protein, or stored in **ferritin**. Bilirubin is a brown/yellow compound which is excreted in the bile. An increased rate of haemoglobin breakdown results in excess bilirubin, which stains the tissues (**jaundice**).

Haemoglobin

Haemoglobin has four subunits, each containing a polypeptide **globin** chain and an iron-containing porphyrin, **haem**. Haem is synthesized from succinic acid and glycine, and contains one atom of iron in the **ferrous** state (Fe^{2+}). One molecule of haemoglobin has therefore four atoms of iron, and binds four molecules of O_2. There are several types of haemoglobin, relating to the globin chains. The haem moiety is unchanged. Adult haemoglobin (Hb A) has two α and two β chains. Fetal haemoglobin (Hb F) has two γ chains in place of the β chains, and a high affinity for O_2. There are several **haemoglobinopathies** due to abnormal haemoglobins.

Sickle cell anaemia is the most important and occurs in 10% of the black population. It is caused by substitution of one glutamic acid by valine in the β chain; the resulting haemoglobin is Hb S. At a low Po_2 Hb S gels, causing deformation (*sickling*) of the erythrocyte. The cell is less flexible and prone to fragmentation, and there is an increased rate of erythrocyte breakdown by macrophages. The Hb S variant is inherited in a mendelian fashion. Heterozygous offspring with less than 40% HB S normally have no symptoms (**sickle cell trait**). Homozygous offspring with more than 70% HB S develop full **sickle cell anaemia**. There are acute episodes of pain relating to blockage of blood vessels, congestion of the liver and spleen with red cells, and commonly leg ulcers.

Thalassaemia is caused by a defect in synthesis of either the α- or β-globin chains. Several genes are involved. In β thalassaemia there are either fewer or no β chains available. The α chains therefore bind to γ (Hb F) or δ chains (Hb A_2). Thalassaemia major (severe β thalassaemia) has high levels of Hb A_2 and Hb F, and severe anaemia. The liver and spleen are enlarged and bone expansion causes typical features. Regular transfusions are required, leading to iron overload. In heterozygous β thalassaemia minor there are no symptoms, although HB A_2 is elevated and erythrocytes are **microcytic** and **hypochromic**, i.e. **mean cell volume** (MCV), **mean cell haemoglobin content** (MCH) and **mean cell haemoglobin concentration** (MCHC) are reduced. In α **thalassaemia** there are fewer or no α chains. In the latter case the haem binds four γ chains (Hb Barts), and does not bind O_2. Infants have huge spleens and livers and oedema (**hydrops fetalis**), and do not survive. When some α chains are present, patients surviving as adults may produce some Hb H (four β chains); this precipitates in the red cells which are then destroyed in the spleen, and this is therefore enlarged.

Anaemia

Some anaemias result from simple blood loss (haemorrhage, heavy menstruation) or chronic disease (e.g. infection, tumours, renal failure). When the cells have an otherwise normal MCV and MCH, the condition is termed **normocytic normochromic** anaemia.

Aplastic anaemia results from an aplastic (nonfunctional) bone marrow and causes **pancytopenia** (reduced red, white and platelet cell count). It is dangerous but uncommon. It can be caused by certain chemicals and drugs (particularly anticancer drugs), radiation, infections (e.g. viral hepatitis, TB) and pregnancy, where it has a 90% mortality. There is a rare inherited condition, **Fanconi's anaemia** which gives rise to a defect in stem cell production and differentiation. Clinical signs include anaemia, bleeding and infections. The condition is variable, and can show either spontaneous remission or gradual and persistent deterioration. Transfusions can be used for maintenance, but long-term treatment may require a bone marrow transplant.

Haemolytic anaemia results from an excessive rate of erythrocyte destruction, and thus causes jaundice. It is associated with blood transfusion mismatch, **haemolytic anaemia of the newborn** (see Chapter 8), abnormal erythrocyte fragility and haemoglobins, and several other disorders including autoimmune, liver and hereditary diseases.

In **hereditary haemolytic anaemia** (familial spherocytosis) erythrocytes have a more spheroid appearance, are more fragile, and more rapidly destroyed in the spleen. It is relatively common, affecting 1 in 5000 Caucasians. Jaundice is common but not invariable at birth, and may appear after several years. Patients may develop aplastic anaemia after infections, and **megaloblastic anaemia** from folate deficiency as a result of high bone marrow activity. Removal of the spleen is normally recommended.

Megaloblastic anaemia: Maturation of the normoblast requires **vitamin B_{12}** (cyanocobalamin) and **folate**, which is commonly given in pregnancy with iron. A reduction in vitamin B_{12} or folate leads to the formation of unusually large normoblasts (**megaloblasts**), which mature as **macrocytes**. These have a large MCV and MCH, although MCHC is normal. The number of red cells is greatly reduced, and the rate of destruction increased. **Folate deficiency** is mostly related to poor diet, in particular in the old or poor. Alcoholism also impairs utilization. Certain anticonvulsant drugs (e.g. phenytoin) have an antifolate action. **Pernicious anaemia** is caused by vitamin B_{12} deficiency as there is defective absorption from the gut. B_{12} is transported across the ileum as a complex with **intrinsic factor**, which is produced by the gastric mucosa. Damage to the gastric mucosa results in pernicious anaemia. B_{12} deficiency can also occur in strict vegans.

Iron deficiency: The daily requirement for **iron** in the diet is small, as the body has an efficient recycling system. It is increased when there is significant blood loss. As a result of menstrual blood loss women have a higher requirement for dietary iron than men. This is increased during pregnancy. **Iron deficiency** causes defective haemoglobin formation and a **microcytic hypochromic** anaemia.

7 Haemostasis and thrombosis

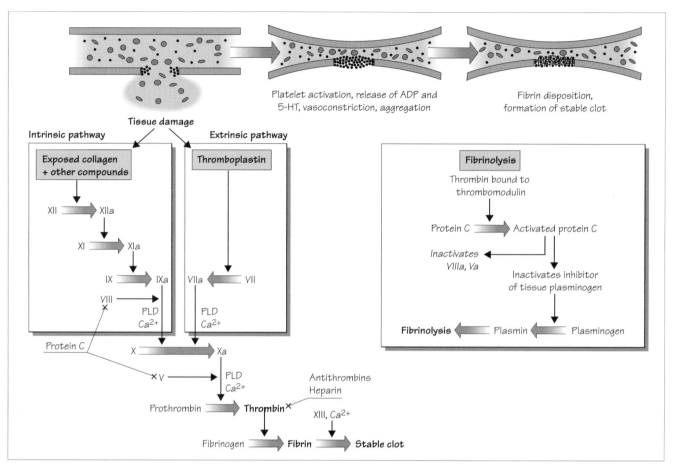

7.1

Haemostasis
Initial response
Damage to the vessel wall or endothelium exposes collagen to the blood. Platelets stick to collagen and activate, releasing **serotonin** (5-HT) and **ADP**. 5-HT is a powerful vasoconstrictor, and local vessels constrict, reducing flow to the injured area. This response is a rapid and effective method of limiting blood loss, but it can only be maintained temporarily. If a clot is prevented from forming (by wiping every 15 s), the period before flow stops is a measure of the effectiveness of this initial response (**bleeding time**), and is normally 2–6 min.

Formation of the blood clot
ADP from activated platelets causes others to activate, put out pseudopodia, and become sticky. More stick to those adhering to the damaged area, resulting in clumping (**platelet aggregation**). The clump grows to a soft **platelet plug** that prevents further blood loss. This is then reinforced with **fibrin**, which traps platelets and blood cells. A complex **cascade** of factors is required for fibrin deposition (see lower left of Fig. 7.1).

Deposition of fibrin
Fibrin is formed from **fibrinogen**, a soluble plasma protein. The protease enzyme **thrombin** cleaves fibrinogen, leaving sticky and insoluble **fibrin monomers**. In the presence of **factor XIII** and Ca^{2+} the monomers polymerize, creating a **stable clot**. Retraction of platelet pseudopodia subsequently causes the clot to contract to ~40% of its original size, becoming tougher and more elastic. Retraction assists repair by drawing the edges of the wound together.

Activation of thrombin
Thrombin is not present in plasma, but is produced when **prothrombin** is activated by **factor X**. This requires Ca^{2+}, **factor V**, and phospholipids (PLD). Two pathways lead to the activation of factor X. In the **extrinsic pathway**, damaged tissues release **thromboplastin**; this, in combination with **factor VII**, directly activates factor X. The time taken for clotting to occur following the addition of thromboplastin to plasma (fibrinogen and Ca^{2+} in excess) is the **prothrombin time**, and this is normally ~14 s. The prothrombin time is

prolonged when prothrombin or factors V, VII and X are deficient.

The **intrinsic pathway** takes minutes for completion. **Factor XII** is activated by exposed collagen and other material following tissue damage. It is activated *in vitro* by negative charges (e.g. glass). A cascade results in the activation of factor X, which requires Ca^{2+} and phospholipids (Fig. 7.1).

The **clotting cascade** is an amplifier. A small stimulus results in a large amount of fibrin. The initial processes take minutes, whereas activation of thrombin and subsequent fibrin deposition is over in seconds. Thus when blood is placed in glass, there is a delay of 5–10 min before the clot suddenly forms (**clotting time**). Formation of the clot all at once is important for haemostasis. In **haemophilia** the clot forms slowly, and is ineffective.

Dissolution of the clot and inhibitors of clotting

The clot is destroyed by the breakdown of fibrin (**fibrinolysis**). Fibrin is broken down by **plasmin**. This is formed from **plasminogen** in the plasma by thrombin and **plasminogen activators**. Fibrinolysis is much slower than clotting. Plasminogen activators are released from damaged tissues, and include **urokinase**.

It is important that clots do not form inappropriately. Circulating protease inhibitors (**antithrombins**) inhibit thrombin and other factors. **Heparin** is a sulphated polysaccharide derived from **mast cells**, which in combination with antithrombin III is a powerful thrombin inhibitor. **Prostacyclin** and **nitric oxide** from the endothelium reduce platelet aggregation. Endothelial cells express **thrombomodulin**, which binds thrombin. This complex activates **protein C**, which with its cofactor **protein S** inactivates factors V and VIII. Protein C also inactivates an inhibitor of plasminogen activator, and so promotes fibrinolysis.

Defects in haemostasis

There are several hereditary **haemophilias** caused by lack of clotting factors. **Clotting time** is prolonged, but **bleeding time** is normal. The most common is **haemophilia A**, where factor VIII is deficient. This is sex linked to the male. **Christmas disease** is a deficiency in factor IX. **Vitamin K** is required by the liver for the production of prothrombin and factors VII, IX and X. It is obtained from intestinal bacteria and food, and disorders of fat absorption can result in vitamin K deficiency and defective clotting. The prothrombin time is prolonged. **Purpura** is associated with easy bruising and spontaneous haemorrhages in the skin and mucus membranes. It is caused by defective haemostatic vasoconstriction, and the bleeding time is prolonged. Some types of purpura are associated with a reduced platelet production (**thrombocytopenia**). The clotting time may be only slightly prolonged, but the clot is soft and does not retract, providing a less effective plug.

Thrombosis

Thrombosis is inappropriate activation of haemostasis that causes formation of a clot (**thrombus**) inside a blood vessel. This can cause occlusion, and in a critical artery is dangerous (e.g. coronary, cerebral). The principal danger from venous thrombi is **embolization**, when they dislodge and are carried elsewhere in the circulation. This can result in **pulmonary embolism**, a major cause of death.

Three main factors predispose to thrombosis, and are referred to as **Virchow's triad**. They are: (i) *damage to the endothelium*; (ii) *poor or turbulent blood flow*; and (iii) *hypercoagulability*. (i) is the most important cause for arterial clots, whereas (ii) and (iii) are more important for venous clots. Damage to the endothelium can lead to clot formation in the absence of other factors. **Myocardial infarction** and valve disease often lead to **endocardial damage**, and are associated with a high risk of thrombosis. **Atheromatous plaques** also predispose to thrombosis. Turbulent blood flow or haemodynamic stress (e.g. hypertension) can cause endothelial injury. Poor blood flow (**stasis**) is a major cause of thrombosis in the venous circulation, and in the **atrium** following atrioventricular (AV) valve stenosis (see Chapter 48). Stasis allows platelets to contact the vessel wall, and activated clotting factors can accumulate because they are not washed away by fresh blood. It also allows unimpeded formation of thrombi.

Hypercoagulability can occur in several genetic and acquired diseases. A high platelet count (**thrombocytosis**) will increase the likelihood of thrombosis. Thrombosis can also result from a defect in factor V (**Leiden's mutation**) that prevents its inactivation by protein C. This is a risk factor for oral contraceptives. Deficiencies in protein C, protein S and antithrombin III are also important in promoting thrombosis.

Once formed, a thrombus may be modified. Fibrinolysis can cause **dissolution**, accumulation of more fibrin and platelets can cause **propagation**. If the thrombus does not dissolve, it may over time be invaded by endothelial and smooth muscle cells, in conjunction with fibrosis (**organization**). Channels may develop through the thrombus (**recanalization**), allowing blood to reflow. The thrombus may eventually be incorporated into the vessel wall.

Anticoagulants

Ca^{2+} is required at several points in the clotting process. Blood for storage can be mixed with **chelating agents** which bind Ca^{2+}. These include citrate, oxalate, and EDTA. Other agents are used for **anticoagulant therapy** *in vivo*. **Heparin** is rapidly acting, and lasts for some hours. **Vitamin K antagonists,** such as **warfarin** and dicoumarol, inhibit the production of prothrombin, and only work *in vivo*. Although slow in onset, they can be effective for days. Low-dose aspirin inhibits platelet aggregation by blocking cyclooxygenase, hence altering the balance between prostacyclin and thromboxane A_2, which causes platelet activation. Anticoagulant therapy is discussed in Chapters 39 and 41.

8 Blood groups and transfusions

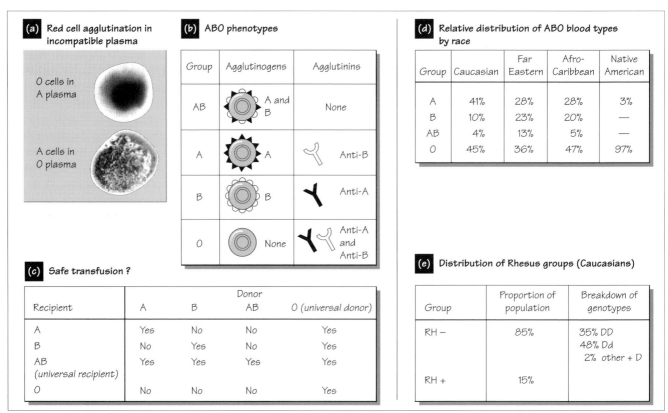

(a) Red cell agglutination in incompatible plasma

O cells in A plasma

A cells in O plasma

(b) ABO phenotypes

Group	Agglutinogens	Agglutinins
AB	A and B	None
A	A	Anti-B
B	B	Anti-A
O	None	Anti-A and Anti-B

(c) Safe transfusion?

Recipient	Donor			
	A	B	AB	O (universal donor)
A	Yes	No	No	Yes
B	No	Yes	No	Yes
AB (universal recipient)	Yes	Yes	Yes	Yes
O	No	No	No	Yes

(d) Relative distribution of ABO blood types by race

Group	Caucasian	Far Eastern	Afro-Caribbean	Native American
A	41%	28%	28%	3%
B	10%	23%	20%	—
AB	4%	13%	5%	—
O	45%	36%	47%	97%

(e) Distribution of Rhesus groups (Caucasians)

Group	Proportion of population	Breakdown of genotypes
RH −	85%	35% DD 48% Dd 2% other + D
RH +	15%	

8.1

Blood groups

If samples of blood from different individuals are mixed together, some combinations result in red cells sticking together as clumps (Fig. 8.1a). This is called **agglutination**, and occurs when the **blood groups** are incompatible. It is caused when antigens (or **agglutinogens**) on the red cell membrane react with specific antibodies (or **agglutinins**) in the plasma. If the quantity (or **titre**) of antibodies is sufficiently high, they bind to their antigens on several red cells and glue the cells together, which then rupture (**haemolyse**). If this occurs following a blood transfusion it can lead to anaemia and other serious complications. The most important blood groups are the **ABO system** and **Rh (Rhesus)** groups.

The ABO system

The ABO system consists of four blood groups: A, B, AB and O. The precise group depends on the presence or absence of two antigens, A and B, on the red cells, and their respective antibodies, α and β, in the plasma (Fig. 8.1b). The A and B antigens on red cells are mostly glycolipids that differ in respect of their terminal sugar. The antigens are also found as glycoproteins in other tissues, including salivary glands, pancreas, lungs and testes, and in saliva and semen.

Group A blood contains the A antigen and β antibody, and group B the B antigen and α antibody. Group AB has both A and B antigens, but neither antibody. Group O blood contains neither antigen, but both α and β antibodies. Group A blood cannot therefore be transfused into people of group B, or vice versa, because antibodies in the recipient react with their respective antigens on the donor red cells and cause agglutination (Fig. 8.1c). As people of group AB have neither α nor β antibodies in the plasma, they can be transfused with blood from any group, and are called **universal recipients**. Group O red cells have neither antigen, and can therefore be transfused into any patient. People of group O are therefore called **universal donors**. Although group O blood contains both antibodies, this can normally be disregarded as they are diluted during transfusion and are bound and neutralized by free A or B antigens in the recipient's plasma. If large or repeated transfusions are required, blood of the same group is used.

Inheritance of ABO blood groups

The expression of A and B antigens is determined genetically. A and B allelomorphs (alternative gene types) are dominant, and O recessive. Therefore AO (**heterozygous**) and AA (**homozygous**) genotypes both have group A phenotypes. An AB genotype produces both antigens, and is thus group AB. The proportion of each blood group varies according to race (Fig. 8.1d), although group O is most common (35–50%). Native Americans are almost exclusively group O.

Rh groups

In ~85% of the population the red cells have a D antigen on the membrane (Fig. 8.1e). Such people are called Rh+ (Rhesus positive), while those who lack the antigen are Rh–. Unlike ABO antigens, the D antigen is not found in other tissues. The antibody to D antigen (**anti-D agglutinin**) is not normally found in the plasma of Rh– individuals, but sensitization and subsequent antibody production occurs if a relatively small amount of Rh+ blood is introduced. This can result from transfusion, or when an Rh– mother has an Rh+ child, and fetal red blood cells enter the maternal circulation during birth. Occasionally fetal cells may cross the placenta earlier in the pregnancy.

Inheritance of Rh groups

The gene corresponding to the D antigen is also called D, and is dominant. When D is absent from the chromosome, its place is taken by the allelomorph of D called d, which is recessive. Individuals who are homozygous and heterozygous for D will be Rh+. About 50% of the population are heterozygous for D, and ~35% homozygous. Blood typing for Rh groups is routinely performed for prospective parents to determine the likelihood of **haemolytic disease** in the offspring.

Haemolytic disease of the newborn

Most pregnancies with Rh– mothers and Rh+ fetuses are normal, but in some cases a severe reaction may occur. Anti-D antibody in the mother's blood can cross the placenta and agglutinate fetal red cells expressing D antigen. The titre of antibody is generally too low to be of consequence during a first pregnancy with a Rh+ fetus, but it can be dangerously increased during subsequent pregnancies, or if the mother was previously sensitized with Rh+ blood. Agglutination of the fetal red cells and consequent haemolysis can result in anaemia and other complications. This is known as **haemolytic disease of the newborn** or **erythroblastosis fetalis**. The haemoglobin released is broken down to bilirubin, which in excess results in **jaundice** (yellow staining of the tissues). If the degree of agglutination and anaemia is severe, the fetus develops severe jaundice and is grossly oedematous (**hydrops fetalis**), and often dies *in utero* or shortly after birth.

Prevention and treatment: In previously unsensitized mothers sensitization can be prevented by treatment with anti-D immunoglobulin after birth. This destroys any fetal Rh+ red cells in the maternal circulation before sensitization of the mother can occur. If haemolytic disease is evident in the fetus or newborn, the Rh+ blood can be replaced by Rh– blood immediately after birth. By the time the newborn has regenerated its own Rh+ red cells, the anti-D antibody from the mother will have been reduced to safe levels. Phototherapy is commonly used for jaundice, as light converts bilirubin to a more rapidly eliminated compound.

Other blood groups

Although there are other bloods groups, these are of little clinical importance, as humans rarely develop antibodies to the respective antigens. They may, however, be of importance in medicolegal situations, e.g. determination of paternity. An example is the MN group, which is a product of two genes (M and N). A person can therefore be MM, MN or NN, each genome coming from one parent. As with the other groups, analysis of the respective parties' genomes can only determine that the man is *not* the father.

Effects of mismatched blood transfusions

When the recipient of a blood transfusion has a significant plasma titre of α, β or anti-D antibodies, donor red cells expressing the respective antigen will rapidly agglutinate and haemolyse (**haemolytic transfusion reaction**). If the subsequent accumulation of bilirubin is sufficiently large, **haemolytic jaundice** develops. In severe cases renal failure may develop. Antibodies in the donor blood are rarely problematical, as they are diluted and removed in the recipient.

Blood storage

Blood is stored for transfusions at 4°C in the presence of an agent that chelates free Ca^{2+} to prevent clotting, for example citrate (see Chapter 7). Even under these conditions the red cells deteriorate, although they last much longer in the presence of glucose, which provides a metabolic substrate. The cell membrane Na^+ pump works more slowly in the cold, with the result that Na^+ enters the cell, and K^+ leaves. This causes water to move into the cell so that it swells, and becomes more spherocytic. On prolonged storage the cells become fragile, and **haemolyse** (fragment) easily. Neither leucocytes nor platelets survive storage well, and disappear within a day of transfusion. Blood banks normally remove all the donor agglutinins (antibodies), although for small transfusions these would be sufficiently diluted to be of no threat. Great care is now taken to screen potential donors for blood-borne diseases (e.g. hepatitis, HIV).

9 Membrane potential, ion channels and pumps

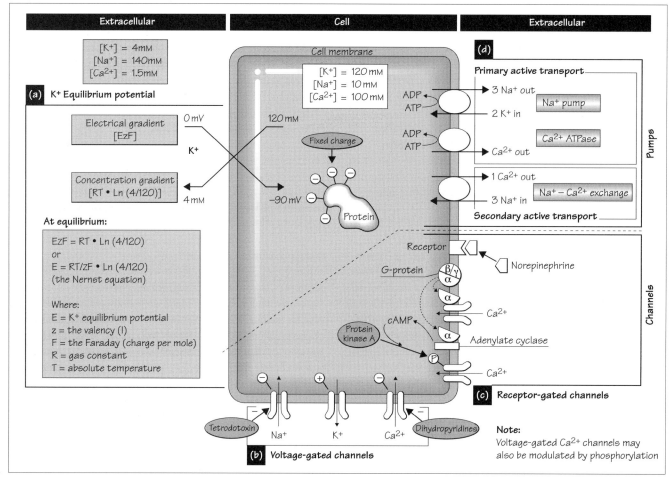

9.1

The cell membrane is composed of a lipid bilayer that has an intrinsically low permeability to charged ions. Spanning the bilayer, however, are a variety of structures through which ions can enter or leave the cell. **Ion channels** allow specific ions to move **passively**, as though through a pore. By contrast, **ion pumps** use energy to **actively transport** ions across the membrane, normally *against* the concentration gradient. Ion channels and pumps are fundamental to cell function. They regulate the ionic gradients across the cell membrane, and determine membrane potential.

The resting membrane potential

At rest, most active ion channels are of a type selective for K+, so that the membrane is more permeable to K+ than other ions. Membranes with this property are called **semipermeable**. The cell contains large negatively charged molecules (e.g. proteins) that cannot cross the membrane. The presence of fixed negative charges attracts positively charged ions. As the membrane is most permeable to K+, this leads to an accumulation of K+ within the cell. However, the *electrical* forces attracting K+ into the cell are then counterbalanced by the increased *concentration gradient*, which tends to drive K+ out of the cell. An equilibrium is reached when these two opposing forces exactly balance. In cardiac muscle cells this occurs when intracellular [K+] is ~120 mM for an extracellular [K+] of ~4 mM. The opposing effect of the concentration gradient means that slightly fewer positive charges (in this case K+ ions) move into the cell than there are intracellular negative charges (e.g. proteins). The inside of the cell is therefore negatively charged compared to the outside (*charge separation*), and as a result a potential develops across the membrane. If the membrane was only permeable to K+, the potential at equilibrium would be defined entirely by the concentration gradient for K+ across the membrane. This is the **K+ equilibrium potential**, and it can be calculated from the **Nernst equation** (Fig. 9.1a).

The actual **resting membrane potential** (RMP) is less negative than the theoretical K+ equilibrium potential. This is because other ions (e.g. Na$^+$) can also cross the membrane, although the membrane permeability for these ions is much less than that for K$^+$. Unlike K$^+$, Na$^+$ has a concentration gradient that is far from equilibrium, as a result of the activity of the **Na$^+$ pump** (Na$^+$–K$^+$ ATPase). This pumps three Na$^+$ ions out of the cell in exchange for two K$^+$ ions into the cell, using ATP as an energy source. As a result intracellular [Na$^+$] is low (~10 mM), even though extracellular [Na$^+$] is high (~140 mM). The equilibrium potential for Na$^+$ (the potential at which electrical and concentration gradient forces would be exactly balanced) is therefore very positive (> +65 mV).

The RMP in a cardiac muscle cell from a ventricle is approximately –90 mV, close to the K$^+$ equilibrium potential. This attracts Na$^+$ ions into the cell. Whereas this inward electrical attraction is balanced in the case of K$^+$ by the *outward* K$^+$ concentration gradient (see above), the concentration gradient for Na$^+$ is inward due to the Na$^+$ pump. Thus both concentration and electrical forces draw Na$^+$ *into* the cell, and the **electrochemical gradient** (the net effect of concentration and electrical forces) is inward. The amount of Na$^+$ actually entering the cell is limited by the low membrane permeability for Na$^+$, and the continuous action of the Na$^+$ pump as it pumps Na$^+$ out. An equivalent situation is apparent for Ca^{2+}, as the Ca^{2+} concentration gradient at rest is ~1.5 mM outside, ~100 nM inside. The small leak of Na$^+$ into the cell causes an inward **background current (I$_b$)** and slight depolarization, so that RMP is less negative than predicted from the K$^+$ equilibrium potential.

Ion channels and gating

There are many channel types, each of which tends to be selective for a particular ion. When a channel is open ions will move passively down their electrochemical gradient. As ions are charged, this causes an electrical current (*ionic current*). Positive ions entering the cell cause an **inward current** and depolarization. Conventionally current caused by outward movement of negative charge (e.g. Cl$^-$) is also called inward, as it has the same effect. During excitation in cardiac and smooth muscle cells, channels mediating the influx of Na$^+$ or Ca^{2+} are opened and the cell depolarizes. The transition of a channel between **closed** and **open** states is called **gating**.

Voltage-gated channels

Voltage-gated channels (VGCs) are gated by membrane potential (Fig. 9.1b). Voltage-gated Na$^+$ and Ca^{2+} channels are activated by depolarization, and are **time dependent**: once opened, they start to **inactivate** immediately. Inactivated channels do not allow the passage of ions. However, they are not in the *closed* state, as they cannot be reopened. This can only happen once they have moved to the true closed state, which does not occur until the membrane potential returns to resting levels. Thus ion flux through VGCs increases rapidly during depolarization, but then falls off at a rate that depends on how fast that type of channel inactivates.

Receptor-gated channels

Receptor-gated channels (RGCs) open when a hormone or neurotransmitter (e.g. norepinephrine) binds to a receptor (Fig. 9.1c). This may involve direct action via **G-proteins** (*GTP binding proteins*) or indirect action via second messenger systems such as cyclic AMP. Cyclic AMP phosphorylates channel proteins, and apart from directly gating some RGCs, can also *modify* the function of channels such as voltage-gated Ca^{2+} channels. Other channel types are gated by *intracellular* factors such as [Ca^{2+}] or [ATP].

Channel activity can both be controlled *by*, and exert an important influence *on*, the membrane potential. An important example is the relationship between membrane potential and voltage-activated Ca^{2+} channels in cardiac muscle and vascular smooth muscle. Depolarization causes channels to open, allowing Ca^{2+} to enter the cell and initiate contraction. In cardiac muscle, the initial depolarization is caused by opening of Na$^+$ channels and initiation of an **action potential**.

Ion pumps and exchangers (Fig. 9.1d)

Whereas movement of ions through channels is passive, ion pumps use energy to pump against the electrochemical gradient. They are primarily concerned with the regulation of cytosolic ion concentrations rather than cell signalling. An important example is the Na$^+$ pump. Pumps that use ATP are referred to as **primary active transport** processes, and another example is the Ca^{2+} ATPase that pumps cytosolic Ca^{2+} into intracellular stores (see Chapters 11, 12). Several other pumps or exchangers use the Na$^+$ electrochemical gradient (maintained by the Na$^+$ pump) as an energy source, and are referred to as **secondary active transport** processes. Na$^+$ binds to the pump and moves down its electrochemical gradient into the cell, effectively twisting the pump so that ions bound on the inside of the membrane are transported out, rather in the way that a water wheel works. Such secondary transport processes include the **Na$^+$–H$^+$ exchanger**, which removes H$^+$ from the cell and helps to control intracellular pH, and the **Na$^+$–Ca^{2+} exchanger**, in which three Na$^+$ ions are exchanged for one Ca^{2+} ion. Inhibitors of the Na$^+$ pump (e.g. **digoxin**) will indirectly inhibit these processes by reducing the Na$^+$ gradient. Pumps are stimulated by the concentrations of their respective ions, although their activity may be modulated by second-messenger-mediated phosphorylation.

Relationship between ion pumps and membrane potential

Some pumps transport unequal amounts of charge across the sarcolemma, e.g. the Na$^+$ pump (3 Na$^+$ to 2 K$^+$) and the Na$^+$–Ca^{2+} exchanger (3 Na$^+$ to 1 Ca^{2+}). Such pumps cause a small but significant ionic current that can affect the membrane potential, and are therefore called **electrogenic**. Electrogenic pumps will themselves be affected by the membrane potential; this is of particular relevance to the Na$^+$–Ca^{2+} exchanger during the cardiac muscle action potential (see Chapters 10, 11).

Electrophysiology of cardiac muscle and the origin of the heart beat

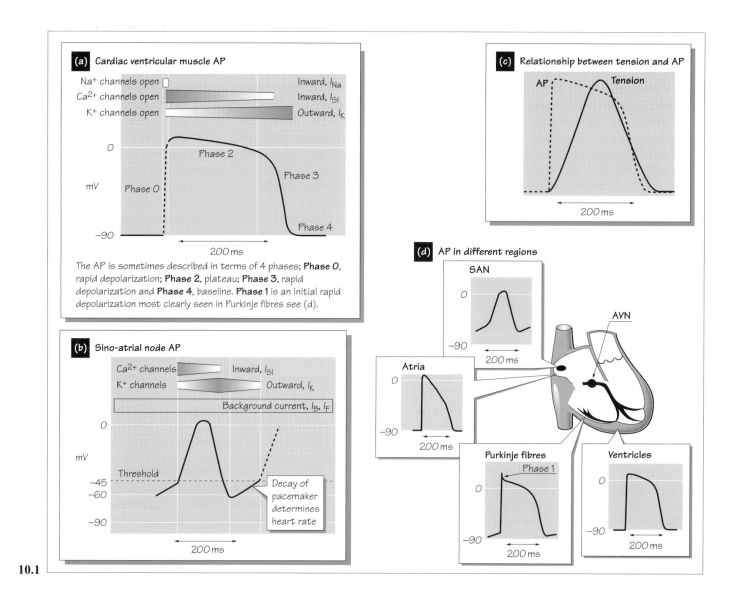

The AP is sometimes described in terms of 4 phases; **Phase 0**, rapid depolarization; **Phase 2**, plateau; **Phase 3**, rapid depolarization and **Phase 4**, baseline. **Phase 1** is an initial rapid depolarization most clearly seen in Purkinje fibres see (d).

10.1

An action potential (AP) is the transient depolarization of a cell as a result of activity of ion channels. The cardiac AP is considerably longer than those occuring in nerve or skeletal muscle (~300 ms vs ~1–3 ms). This is due to the presence of a **plateau phase** in cardiac muscle, which lasts for 200–300 msec.

Ventricular muscle action potential (Fig. 10.1a)

Initiation of the action potential

At rest, the membrane is most permeable to K+ ions and the **resting potential** is primarily dependent on the K+ concentration gradient (see Chapter 9). An AP is initiated when the membrane is depolarized to a **threshold potential** (~–65 mV). The initial depolarization results from transmission from an adjacent cell through **intercalated disks**. At the threshold potential the inward current caused by entry of Na+ through voltage-gated Na+ channels (I_{Na}) becomes large enough to overcome the outward current through K+ channels, and thus causes further depolarization. This in turn activates more Na+ channels. The depolarization thus becomes self generating, and so results in a very rapid upstroke (phase 0; ~500 V/s). At this point the membrane is more permeable to Na+ than K+ because of the open Na+ channels. The Na+ concentration gradient therefore becomes the major determinant of membrane potential, and the cell moves *towards* the equilibrium potential for Na+ (~+65 mV) (see Chapter 9). It does not reach this potential both because it is limited by the existing K+ permeability, and because of rapid **inactivation** (shutting) of the Na+ channels. The Na+ channels cannot be reactivated until the potential becomes more negative than ~-65 mV. Therefore another AP cannot be initiated until the cell repolarizes *to at least* this potential (**absolute refractory period**). At slightly more negative potentials some Na^+ channels reactivate, allowing an AP to be initiated by a sufficiently large stimulus (**relative refractory period**). All Na^+ channels are reactivated by the time the cell is completely repolarized. The refractory period, and the length of the AP compared to the twitch (Fig. 10.1c) means that, unlike skeletal muscle, cardiac muscle cannot be tetanized.

The plateau phase

At the end of the upstroke, membrane Na^+ permeability returns to its resting value, and in skeletal muscle this results in rapid repolarization. In cardiac muscle however, the membrane potential decays slowly over ~250 ms before a more rapid repolarization phase. This period of slow decay is the **plateau phase** (phase 2), and is primarily due to Ca^{2+} entering the cell via **voltage-sensitive L-type Ca^{2+} channels**, which activate relatively slowly when the membrane potential becomes more positive than ~-35 mV. The resultant Ca^{2+} current (**slow inward current** or I_{SI}), coupled with a reduced K^+ outward current, is sufficient to slow repolarization until the potential falls to ~-20 mV. The length of the plateau is related to slow **inactivation** of Ca^{2+} channels. Ca^{2+} entry during the plateau is vital for contraction; blockers of L-type Ca^{2+} channels (e.g. **dihydropyridines**) reduce force (see Chapter 11).

Repolarization (phase 3)

At the end of the plateau the K^+ outward current becomes dominant, and membrane potential returns to its resting level (phase 4). Several types of K^+ channel contribute to repolarization. Factors that influence outward current will affect the rate of repolarization, and hence the length of AP.

Role of Na^+–Ca^{2+} exchange during the action potential

In the early stages of the plateau, when it is most positive and the Na^+ electrochemical gradient is therefore at its smallest, the Na^+–Ca^{2+} exchanger may be reversed, and contribute to the inward movement of Ca^{2+}. As the plateau decays and becomes more negative the Na^+ electrochemical gradient increases, and the Na^+–Ca^{2+} exchanger returns to its usual function of expelling Ca^{2+}. The resulting influx of Na^+ ions causes an inward current that may slow repolarization and reduce the rate of decay of the plateau, thus lengthening the AP.

Sinoatrial node and the origin of the heart beat

The AP of the **sinoatrial node** (SAN, Fig. 10.1b) differs in several important aspects from that of the ventricle. The upstroke in the SAN is much slower than in the ventricle. This is because there are no functional Na^+ channels, and depolarization is caused by Ca^{2+} entry via slowly activating Ca^{2+} channels. The slower upstroke leads to slower conduction from cell to cell (see Chapter 15). This is of particular importance in the **atrioventricular node** (AVN), which has a similar AP to the SAN.

In direct contrast to the ventricle, the SAN has an unstable resting potential which decays from ~-60 mV to a threshold potential of ~-40 mV, at which point an AP is initiated. The threshold potential is more positive than that in the ventricle, because voltage-gated Ca^{2+} channels, which underlie the upstroke in the SAN, have a more positive threshold than voltage-gated Na^+ channels, which underlie the upstroke in the ventricle. The rate of decay of the SAN resting potential determines the rate at which APs are generated, and hence heart rate. The resting potential is therefore commonly called the **pacemaker potential**. The pacemaker potential relies on a K^+ outward current that slowly decays with time (I_K), and two relatively stable inward currents, mostly due to the inward movement of Na^+. These are I_b, which is also present in other cardiac cells, and I_f ('*funny*'), which appears to be specific to the SAN. As the outward I_K decays, this allows the contribution from the inward I_f and I_b to become more dominant, and the membrane depolarizes.

Factors that influence these currents alter the slope of the pacemaker and thus heart rate, and are called **chronotropic agents**. The sympathetic neurotransmitter norepinephrine increases heart rate by increasing the slope of the pacemaker, caused by an increase in the size of I_f. It also reduces the length of the AP by increasing the rate of Ca^{2+} entry and hence the slope of the upstroke. The parasympathetic transmitter acetylcholine reduces the slope of the pacemaker, and causes a small hyper-polarization, both of which increase the time required to reach threshold, and reduce heart rate.

Action potentials in other regions of the heart (Fig. 10.1d)

AVN APs are similar to those of the SAN. Atrial muscle has a similar AP to ventricular muscle, although the shape is more triangular. **Purkinje fibres** in the conduction system have a spike at the peak of upstroke (phase 1). This relates to a greater inward Na^+ current and more rapid upstroke, and contributes to faster conduction. The AVN, bundle of His and Purkinje system may also have decaying resting potentials that can act as pacemakers. However, the SAN is normally fastest and predominates. This is called **dominance** or **overdrive suppression**.

Effects of plasma [K^+]

Several conditions increase plasma [K^+] (e.g. renal failure, tissue damage). If it rises above ~5.5 mM (**hyperkalaemia**) there can be serious consequences, as the membrane depolarizes and becomes closer to threshold potential. This can cause dangerous arrhythmias, e.g. ventricular fibrillation, especially where the myocardium is diseased (see Chapter 45). Hyperkalaemia also slows and weakens the AP upstroke due to partial inactivation of Na^+ channels, and slows conduction. Above 8 mM this leads to complete cessation of conduction (**heart block**). Conversely **hypokalaemia** ($< \sim3$ mM [K^+]) hyperpolarizes the membrane, making it more difficult to reach threshold and also affecting conduction. Hypokalaemia is commonly associated with diuretic therapy in heart disease (e.g. Chapter 44).

11 Excitation–contraction coupling in cardiac muscle cells

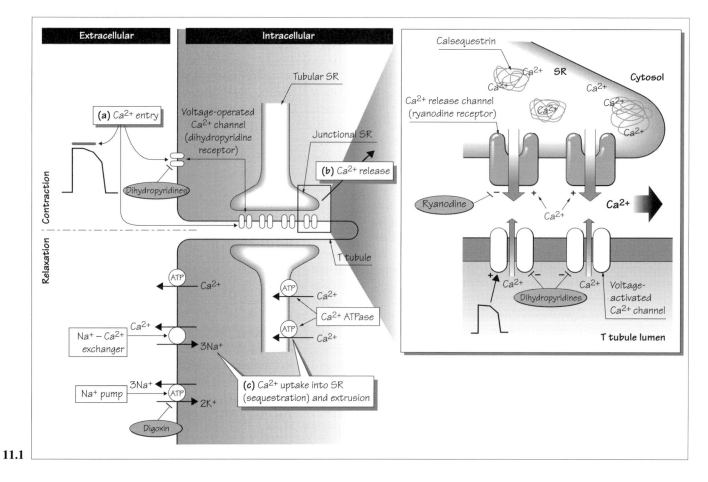

11.1

Cardiac muscle contracts when cytosolic [Ca2+] rises above about 100 nM. This rise in [Ca2+] couples the action potential (AP) to contraction, and the mechanisms involved are referred to as **excitation–contraction coupling**. The relationship between cardiac muscle force and stretch is discussed in Chapter 14. The ability of cardiac muscle to generate force *for any given fibre length* is described as its **contractility**. This depends on cytosolic [Ca2+], and to a lesser extent on factors which affect the Ca2+ sensitivity of the contractile apparatus. The contractility of cardiac muscle is primarily dependent on the way that the cell handles Ca2+.

Initiation of contraction

During the **plateau phase** of the AP Ca2+ enters the cell through **L-type voltage-gated Ca2+ channels** in the **sarcolemma** (muscle cell membrane; Fig. 11.1a). L-type channels are specifically blocked by **dihydropyridines** (e.g. **nifedipine**) and *verapamil*. However, the amount of Ca2+ that enters the cell is less than 20% of that required for the observed rise in cytosolic [Ca2+] ([Ca2+]$_i$). The rest is released from the **sarcoplasmic reticulum** (SR), where it is stored bound to **calsequestrin** (Fig. 11.1b). The

action potential travels into the **T tubules** and during the first 1–2 ms of the plateau Ca2+ enters and causes a small rise in [Ca2+] in the gap between the sarcolemma and the **junctional SR**. This activates **Ca2+-sensitive release channels** in the SR, through which stored Ca2+ floods into the cytoplasm. These channels are sometimes referred to as ryanodine receptors, because they can bind, and be locked into a partially open state, by the drug ryanodine. A rapid increase in [Ca2+]$_i$ occurs over the next 10 ms, and tension starts to develop. This process is called **calcium-induced calcium release**.

The amount of Ca2+ released depends on how much is stored in the SR and the number of release channels activated, and thus the amount of Ca2+ entering across the sarcolemma. *In the absence of external Ca2+ there is no contraction.* Peak [Ca2+]$_i$ normally rises to ~2 μM, although maximum contraction occurs when [Ca2+]$_i$ rises above 10 μM. Cardiac muscle force can therefore be regulated by altering either the amount of Ca2+ entering during the AP, or the amount stored in the SR.

Generation of tension

The physical arrangement of **actin** and **myosin** filaments is discussed in Chapter 2. Force is generated when the myosin heads protruding from the thick filament bind to sites on actin to form **crossbridges**, and drag the actin past in a ratchet fashion, using ATP bound to myosin as an energy source. This is the **sliding filament** or **crossbridge mechanism** of muscle contraction.

Regulation of crossbridge formation

In cardiac muscle, $[Ca^{2+}]_i$ controls crossbridge formation via the regulatory proteins **tropomyosin** and **troponin**. Tropomyosin is a coiled strand which, at rest, lies in the cleft between the two actin chains that form the thin filament helix, and covers the myosin binding sites on the actin. The myosin heads therefore cannot bind, and there is no tension. Troponin is formed from a complex of three smaller globular proteins (**troponin C, I and T**), which is bound to tropomyosin by **troponin T** at intervals of 40 nm. When $[Ca^{2+}]_i$ rises above 100 nM, Ca^{2+} binds to **troponin C** and there is a conformational change involving dissociation of **troponin I** from actin, which allows tropomyosin to shift out of the actin cleft. The binding sites are uncovered, myosin crossbridges form, and tension develops. Tension is related to the number of active crossbridges, and will increase until all troponin C is bound to Ca^{2+} ($[Ca^{2+}]_i > 10 \ \mu M$).

Relaxation mechanisms

When $[Ca^{2+}]_i$ rises above the resting level (~100 nM), ATP-dependent Ca^{2+} pumps (**Ca^{2+}-ATPase**) in the tubular part of the SR are activated, and start to pump Ca^{2+} from the cytosol back into the SR (Fig. 11.1c). As the AP repolarizes and voltage-dependent Ca^{2+} channels inactivate, this mechanism reduces $[Ca^{2+}]_i$ towards resting levels, Ca^{2+} ions dissociate from troponin C, and the muscle relaxes.

If there were no other mechanisms to remove Ca^{2+} from the cell, the size of the SR Ca^{2+} store would gradually increase as more Ca^{2+} enters during each AP. Excess Ca^{2+} is transported out of the cell by the **Na^+–Ca^{2+} exchanger** in the sarcolemma (Fig. 11.1c; see Chapter 9). This uses the inward Na^+ electrochemical gradient as an energy source to pump Ca^{2+} out, and in the process three Na^+ ions enter the cell for each Ca^{2+} ion removed. There are also Ca^{2+}-ATPase pumps in the sarcolemma, but their importance is probably minor. At the end of the AP about 80% of the Ca^{2+} will have been resequestered into the SR, and most of the rest ejected from the cell. The remainder is slowly pumped out during the diastolic interval.

Modulation of cardiac muscle tension

Inotropic agents

Factors that alter the contractility of cardiac muscle are called **inotropic agents**. A positive inotropic agent increases contractility, whereas a negative one decreases it. Most inotropic agents act via mechanisms that regulate $[Ca^{2+}]_i$, although some may alter Ca^{2+} binding to troponin-C. For example, a high plasma $[Ca^{2+}]$ increases contractility by increasing Ca^{2+} entry during the AP.

Norepinephrine from sympathetic nerve endings, and to a lesser extent circulating **epinephrine**, are the most important physiological inotropic agents. They also increase heart rate (positive **chronotropes**; see Chapter 10). Norepinephrine binds to β-adrenoceptors on the sarcolemma, and thus increases cAMP. cAMP-mediated phosphorylation of Ca^{2+} channels increases Ca^{2+} entry during the AP, and elevates $[Ca^{2+}]_i$. Norepinephrine may also activate Ca^{2+} channels directly via G-proteins (see Chapter 9). The rate of Ca^{2+} uptake into the SR, and hence the rate of relaxation, is also increased by norepinephrine, via cAMP-mediated phosphorylation of **phospholamban**, a regulatory protein associated with the Ca^{2+}-ATPase.

Cardiac glycosides such as **digoxin** are specific inhibitors of the **Na^+ pump** and increase cytosolic $[Na^+]$, so reducing the Na^+ gradient across the sarcolemma that drives Na^+–Ca^{2+} exchange. As a result less Ca^{2+} is removed from the cell, and more ends up in the SR. There is therefore more available for release, and peak $[Ca^{2+}]_i$ and tension increases. The clinical use of digoxin is discussed in Chapter 44.

The influence of heart rate

When heart rate increases there is a proportional rise in cardiac muscle force. This phenomenon is known as the **staircase**, **Treppe** or **Bowditch** effect. It can be attributed both to an increase in cytosolic $[Na^{2+}]$ due to the greater frequency of APs, with a consequent inhibition of the Na^+–Ca^{2+} exchanger (see above), and to a decreased diastolic interval over which Ca^{2+} can be extruded from the cell, resulting in more Ca^{2+} in the SR. The relative importance of these mechanisms is unclear.

12 Vascular smooth muscle excitation–contraction coupling

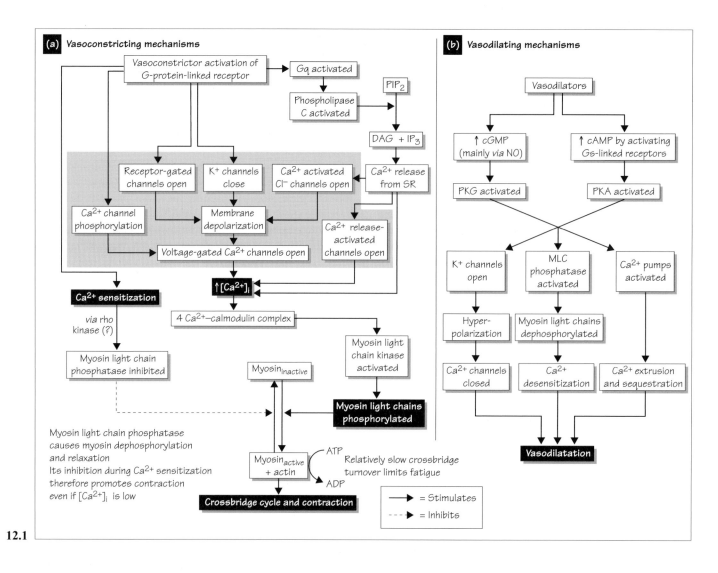

12.1

Vascular smooth muscle (VSM) contraction is, like that of cardiac muscle, controlled by the *intracellular Ca²⁺ concentration* $[Ca^{2+}]_i$. Unlike cardiac muscle cells, however, VSM cells lack troponin and utilize a *myosin-based system* to regulate contraction.

Regulation of contraction by Ca²⁺ and myosin phosphorylation

Vasoconstricting stimuli initiate VSM cell contraction by increasing $[Ca^{2+}]_i$ from its basal level of ~100 nM. Force development is proportional to the increase in $[Ca^{2+}]_i$, with maximal contraction occurring at ~1 μM $[Ca^{2+}]_i$. The rise in $[Ca^{2+}]_i$ promotes its binding to the cytoplasmic regulatory protein **calmodulin**. Once a calmodulin molecule has bound four Ca²⁺ ions, it can activate the enzyme **myosin light-chain kinase** (MLCK). MLCK in turn phosphorylates two 20-kDa subunits (**'light chains'**) contained within the 'head' of each myosin molecule. Phosphorylated

myosin then forms crossbridges with actin, using ATP hydrolysis as an energy source to produce contraction. Actin–myosin interactions during crossbridge cycling are similar to those in cardiac myocytes (see Chapter 11).

The degree of myosin light-chain phosphorylation, which determines crossbridge turnover, is a balance between the activity of MLCK and a **myosin light-chain phosphatase** which dephosphorylates the light chains. Once $[Ca^{2+}]_i$ falls, MLCK activity diminishes and relaxation occurs as light-chain phosphorylation is returned to basal levels by the phosphatase.

VSM cells *in vivo* maintain a tonic level of partial contraction that varies with fluctuations in the vasoconstricting and vasodilating influences to which they are exposed. VSM cells avoid fatigue during prolonged contractions because their rate of ATP consumption is 300-fold lower than that of skeletal muscle fibres. This is possible because the crossbridge cycle is much slower than in striated muscles. The maximum crossbridge cycling rate of smooth muscle during shortening is only about 1/10 of that in striated muscles, as a result of differences in the types of myosin present. In addition, once they have shortened, vascular cells can maintain contraction with an even lower expenditure of ATP because the myosin crossbridges remain attached to actin for a longer time, thus 'locking in' shortening.

Vasoconstricting mechanisms

The binding to receptors of **norepinephrine** and other important vasoconstrictors such as **endothelin, thromboxane A₂, angiotensin II** and **vasopressin** stimulates VSM contraction via common **G-protein-mediated** pathways (Fig. 12.1a).

Ca²⁺ release

Binding of vasoconstrictors to receptors activates the G-protein **Gq**, which stimulates the enzyme **phospholipase C**. Phospholipase C splits the membrane phospholipid phosphatidylinositol 1,4-bisphosphate, generating the second messengers inositol 1,4,5-triphosphate (**IP₃**), and diacylglycerol (**DAG**). IP₃ binds to and opens Ca²⁺ channels on the membrane of the **sarcoplasmic reticulum** (SR). This allows Ca²⁺, which is stored in high concentrations within the SR, to flood out into the cytoplasm and rapidly increase [Ca²⁺]ᵢ. DAG activates **protein kinase C** (PKC).

Effects on ion channels

Vasoconstrictors also cause **membrane depolarization** via several mechanisms. First, the release of SR Ca²⁺ which they initiate opens **Ca²⁺-activated chloride channels** in the plasma membrane. Second, vasoconstrictors may cause depolarization by *inhibiting* the activity of **K⁺ channels**. Third, vasoconstrictors both induce membrane depolarization and Ca²⁺ entry into VSM cells by opening **receptor-gated cation channels**, which allow the influx of both Na⁺ and Ca²⁺ ions.

The membrane depolarization elicited by vasoconstrictors opens **voltage-gated Ca²⁺ channels** similar to those found in cardiac myocytes. With sufficient depolarization, some blood vessels may fire brief Ca²⁺ channel-mediated APs that cause transient contractions. More often, however, blood vessels respond to vasoconstrictors with graded depolarizations, during which sufficient Ca²⁺ influx occurs to cause more sustained contractions.

There is recent evidence that vasoconstrictors can promote Ca²⁺ influx by two additional mechanisms related to pathways described above. First, depletion of Ca²⁺ from the SR due to the action of IP₃ opens a **Ca²⁺ release-activated channel** in the cell membrane which admits Ca²⁺ to the cell. Second, G-protein-linked mechanisms directly enhance the opening of voltage-gated Ca²⁺ channels, probably via channel phosphorylation.

As well as raising [Ca²⁺]ᵢ, vasoconstrictors also promote contraction by a process termed **Ca²⁺ sensitization**. Ca²⁺ sensitization is caused by the inhibition of myosin phosphatase. This increases myosin light-chain phosphorylation, and therefore force development, even with minimal increases in [Ca²⁺]ᵢ and MLCK activity. Recent evidence suggests that phosphatase inhibition may be primarily caused by **rhoA kinase**, an enzyme stimulated by the *ras* type G protein **rhoA**, which is activated by vasoconstrictors. PKC may also contribute to Ca²⁺ sensitization.

The relative importance of the excitatory mechanisms listed above varies between different vasoconstrictors and vascular beds. In resistance arteries depolarization and Ca²⁺ influx through voltage-gated channels are probably most important.

Ca²⁺ removal mechanisms

Several mechanisms serve to remove Ca²⁺ from the cytoplasm. These are continually active, allowing cells both to recover from stimulation and to maintain a low basal [Ca²⁺]ᵢ in the face of the enormous electrochemical gradient tending to drive Ca²⁺ into cells even when they are not stimulated. The **smooth endoplasmic reticulum Ca²⁺-ATPase (SERCA)** pumps Ca²⁺ from the cytoplasm into the SR. This process is referred to as **Ca²⁺ sequestration**. A similar **plasma membrane Ca²⁺-ATPase (PMCA)** pumps Ca²⁺ from the cytoplasm into the extracellular space (**Ca²⁺ extrusion**). Cells also extrude Ca²⁺ via a **Na/Ca antiport** located in the cell membrane, which is similar to that found in cardiac cells (see Chapter 11). The Na/Ca antiport may be localized to areas of the plasma membrane which are approached closely by the sarcoplasmic reticulum, allowing any Ca²⁺ leaking from the SR to be quickly ejected from the cell without causing tension development.

Vasodilator mechanisms

Most vasodilators acting on smooth muscle cells cause relaxation by activating either the cyclic **GMP** (e.g. nitric oxide, ANP)) or cyclic **AMP** (e.g. adenosine, prostacyclin, β receptor agonists) second messenger systems (Fig. 12.1b). Both second messengers activate kinases, which act by phosphorylating overlapping sets of cellular proteins. cGMP activates **cyclic GMP-dependent protein kinase (PKG)**. The mechanisms by which PKG causes relaxation have not been conclusively established. It has been reported, however, that PKG causes hyperpolarization by activating K⁺ channels, and that it stimulates both Ca²⁺ sequestration and extrusion by activating the SERCA and PMCA.

Cyclic AMP exerts its effects via **cyclic AMP-dependent protein kinase (protein kinase A or PKA)**, although high levels of cAMP have also been shown to stimulate PKG. PKA is thought to cause smooth muscle cell relaxation by lowering [Ca²⁺]ᵢ. There is evidence that it does so by stimulating the SERCA, and also by opening **ATP-sensitive (K_ATP)** and **Ca²⁺-activated K⁺ (BK) channels**. This causes membrane hyperpolarization, which inhibits Ca²⁺ influx by switching off voltage-gated Ca²⁺ channels, a fraction of which are open even at the resting membrane potential. Hyperpolarization is additionally reported to inhibit phospholipase C activity, thereby reducing IP₃ production. PKA can also phosphorylate MLCK, thereby inhibiting its activity. The contribution of this mechanism to relaxation under physiological conditions is, however, controversial.

13 Cardiac cycle

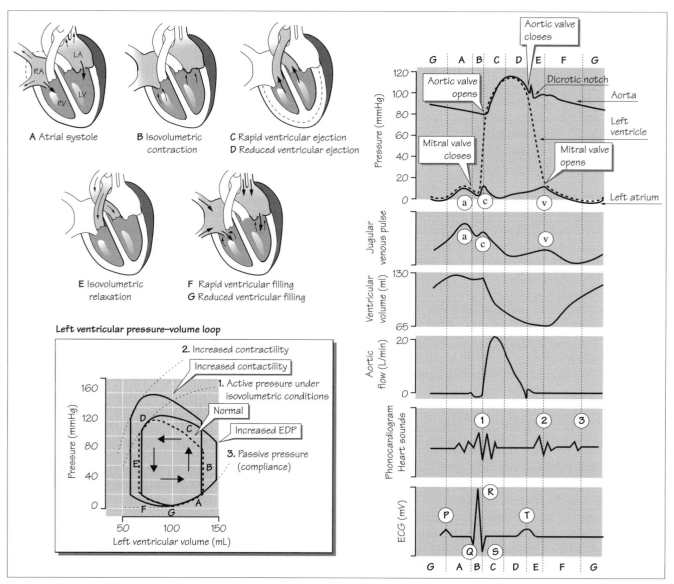

A Atrial systole

B Isovolumetric contraction

C Rapid ventricular ejection
D Reduced ventricular ejection

E Isovolumetric relaxation

F Rapid ventricular filling
G Reduced ventricular filling

Left ventricular pressure–volume loop

2. Increased contractility

Increased contactility

1. Active pressure under isovolumetric conditions

Normal

Increased EDP

3. Passive pressure (compliance)

Aortic valve closes

Aortic valve opens

Dicrotic notch

Aorta

Left ventricle

Mitral valve closes

Mitral valve opens

Left atrium

13.1

The **cardiac cycle** is the sequence of mechanical events that occurs during a single heart beat.

Towards the end of **diastole** (G) all chambers of the heart are relaxed. The valves between the atria and ventricles are open (**AV valves**: right, **tricuspid**; left, **mitral**), because atrial pressure remains slightly greater than ventricular pressure until the ventricles are fully distended. The **pulmonary** and **aortic** (semilunar) **outflow valves** are closed, as pulmonary artery and aortic pressure is greater than ventricular pressure. The cycle begins when the **sinoatrial node** initiates the heart beat.

Atrial systole (A)
Contraction of the atria completes ventricular filling. At rest,

the atria contribute less than 20% of final ventricular volume. The remainder is contributed by venous pressure. The atrial contribution increases as heart rate rises, as diastole shortens and there is less time for ventricular filling. There are no valves between the veins and atria, and some blood regurgitates into the veins. The **a wave** of atrial and venous pressure traces reflects atrial systole. Ventricular volume after filling is known as **end-diastolic volume** (EDV), and is ~120–140 ml. The equivalent pressure (**end-diastolic pressure**, EDP) is less than 10 mmHg, and is higher in the left ventricle than in the right due to the more muscular and therefore stiffer left ventricular wall. EDV is an important determinant of the strength of the subsequent contraction (Starling's Law, see

Chapter 14). Atrial depolarization causes the **P wave** of the ECG.

Ventricular systole

Ventricular contraction causes a sharp rise in ventricular pressure, and the atrioventricular (AV) valves close once this exceeds atrial pressure. Ventricular depolarization is associated with the **QRS complex** of the ECG. During the initial phase of ventricular contraction pressure is less than that in the pulmonary artery and aorta, so the outflow valves remain closed. This is **isovolumetric contraction** (B), as ventricular volume does not change. The increasing pressure causes the AV valves to bulge into the atria, resulting in the small atrial pressure wave (**c wave**).

Ejection

The outflow valves open when pressure in the ventricle exceeds that in the artery. Note that pulmonary artery pressure (~15 mmHg) is considerably less than that in the aorta (~80 mmHg). Flow into the arteries is initially very rapid (**rapid ejection phase**, C), but as contraction wanes ejection is reduced (**reduced ejection phase**, D). Active contraction ceases during the second half of ejection, and the muscle repolarizes. This is associated with the **T wave** of the ECG. Ventricular pressure during the reduced ejection phase is slightly less than that in the artery, but blood continues to flow out of the ventricle because of momentum. Eventually the flow briefly reverses, causing closure of the outflow valve and a small increase in aortic pressure, the **dicrotic notch**.

The amount of blood ejected by the ventricle in one beat is the **stroke volume**, ~70 ml. About 50 ml of blood is therefore left in the ventricle at the end of systole (**end-systolic volume**). The proportion of EDV that is ejected (stroke volume/EDV) is the **ejection fraction**.

Diastole—relaxation and refilling

In the period following closure of the outflow valves the ventricles are rapidly relaxing. Ventricular pressure is still greater than atrial pressure however, and the AV valves remain closed. This is known as **isovolumetric relaxation** (E). During the last two-thirds of systole atrial pressure rises as a result of filling from the veins (**v wave**). When ventricular pressure falls below atrial pressure, the AV valves open, and atrial pressure falls as the ventricles rapidly refill (**rapid ventricular refilling**, F). This is assisted by elastic recoil of the ventricular walls, essentially sucking in the blood. As the ventricles relax completely refilling slows (**reduced refilling**, G). This continues during the last two-thirds of diastole due to venous flow. At rest, diastole is twice the length of systole, but decreases proportionately during exercise and as heart rate increases.

The pressure–volume loop

Ventricular pressure plotted against volume generates a loop (Fig. 13.1). The shape of the loop is affected by the **contractility** (see Chapter 14) and **compliance** ('*stretchiness*') of the ventricle, and factors that alter **refilling** or **ejection** (e.g. CVP, afterload). The upper dashed lines that confine the loops (**1** and **2**) show the pressure that would be generated at any volume if the outflow valves remained closed (Starling curves, see Chapter 14). The bottom line (**3**) shows the passive elastic properties of the ventricle (compliance). If compliance was decreased as a result of fibrotic damage following an infarct, the curve would be steeper. The area of the loop (Δ pressure $\times$ Δ volume) is a measure of work done by the heart during a beat, and is an indicator of cardiac function. A common clinical estimate of **stroke work** is calculated from mean arterial pressure $\times$ stroke volume.

Cardiac auscultation—heart sounds and murmurs

The **first heart sound** (S_1) is low frequency ('lubb'), and associated with closure of the AV valves. These normally close simultaneously, and **splitting** of S_1 may reflect delayed electrical conduction in the left or right bundles of His (see Chapter 15). The **second heart sound** (S_2) is of higher frequency ('dup'), and often splits in young people during inspiration and exercise, reflecting a longer ejection period in the right ventricle. The **third heart sound** (S_3) is associated with rapid refilling, and is most commonly heard in young people. In adults it may represent stiffening of the ventricle. A **fourth heart sound** (S_4) is associated with atrial systole, but is rarely audible except when the EDP is raised. When S_3 and/or S_4 are present, they produce a triple sound similar to a galloping horse, a **'gallop rhythm'**.

Cardiac **murmurs** are caused by turbulent bloodflow. A murmur during the ejection phase is often heard in young people, and is benign. Other murmurs can reflect valve defects (see Chapters 48, 49). In **stenosis** the valve is narrowed, and blood velocity increases. This promotes turbulence and creates a murmur. In **incompetence** the valve leaks blood while closed, and this **regurgitation** is heard as a dull roar. Aortic incompetence leads to a diastolic murmur and softening and prolongation of the second heart sound. A **thrill** is a clear vibration.

The arterial pulse

The peripheral pulse is caused by pressure waves travelling down the arterial tree. The shape of the pulse is modified by the compliance and size of the artery. A stiff artery, as in advancing age or atherosclerosis, results in a sharper pulse. The pulse also becomes sharper as artery size decreases. Reflections back up the artery from points where resistance to flow increases, e.g. where the artery divides, can give rise to further peaks. A small, slowly rising pulse can be caused by stenosis of the aortic valve. Aortic valve incompetence can cause a hard knocking sensation as the pulse pressure falls rapidly after each beat. This is called a **collapsing** or **Corrigan** pulse (see Chapter 48).

The **jugular venous pulse** reflects the right atrial pressure, and has corresponding **a, c** and **v waves** (see above).

14 Control of cardiac output and Starling's Law of the Heart

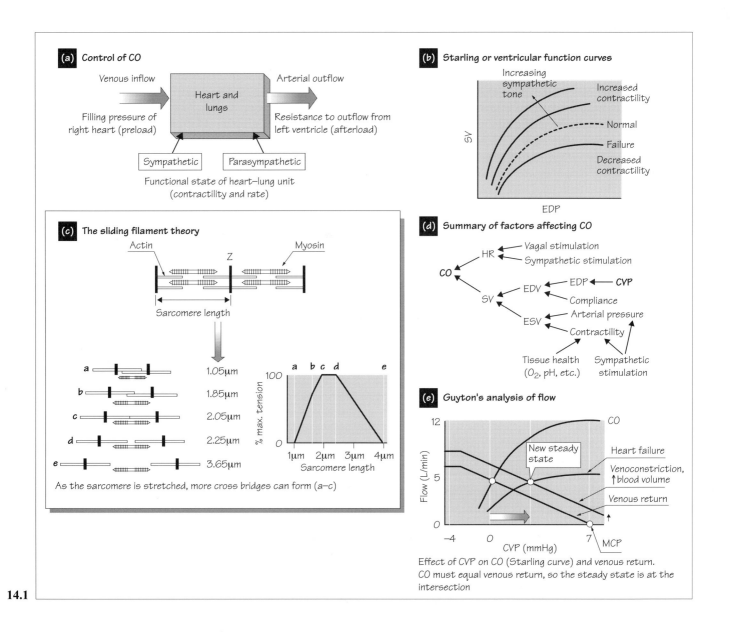

(a) Control of CO

Venous inflow → Heart and lungs → Arterial outflow

Filling pressure of right heart (preload)

Resistance to outflow from left ventricle (afterload)

Sympathetic | Parasympathetic

Functional state of heart–lung unit (contractility and rate)

(b) Starling or ventricular function curves

Increasing sympathetic tone
Increased contractility
Normal
Failure
Decreased contractility

SV
EDP

(c) The sliding filament theory

Actin   Z   Myosin

Sarcomere length

a — 1.05µm
b — 1.85µm
c — 2.05µm
d — 2.25µm
e — 3.65µm

100
% max. tension
0
a b c d   e
1µm 2µm 3µm 4µm
Sarcomere length

As the sarcomere is stretched, more cross bridges can form (a–c)

(d) Summary of factors affecting CO

CO
HR — Vagal stimulation
     — Sympathetic stimulation
SV
  EDV — EDP ← CVP
        Compliance
  ESV — Arterial pressure
        Contractility
Tissue health (O₂, pH, etc.)   Sympathetic stimulation

(e) Guyton's analysis of flow

12
Flow (L/min)
5
0
−4   0   7
CVP (mmHg)

CO
New steady state
Heart failure
Venoconstriction, ↑blood volume
Venous return
MCP

Effect of CVP on CO (Starling curve) and venous return. CO must equal venous return, so the steady state is at the intersection

14.1

Cardiac output (CO) is the volume of blood pumped through the heart per minute, i.e. stroke volume (SV) × heart rate (HR). In a normal 70-kg man cardiac output at rest is about 5 L/min, but during strenuous exercise this can rise to 25 L/min or more.

Control of cardiac output

If the heart and lungs are considered as a unit, it can be seen that only three things can directly influence cardiac output (Fig. 14.1a). These are the filling pressure of the right heart (**preload**), the resistance to outflow from the left ventricle (**afterload**), and the functional state of the heart. The latter includes heart rate and **contractility** (see Chapter 11), which are

modulated by the **sympathetic** and **parasympathetic** nervous systems.

Filling pressure and stroke volume

The amount of blood in the ventricle at the start of systole (**end-diastolic volume**, EDV) depends on the **end-diastolic pressure** (EDP) and the **compliance** of the ventricular wall (how easy it is to inflate). Right ventricular EDP is primarily dependent on **central venous pressure** (CVP). If EDP (and thus EDV) is increased, the force of the next contraction and stroke volume also increases (Fig. 14.1b). This is known as the **Frank–Starling** relationship. The graph relating stroke volume to EDP is called a **Starling** or **ventricular function** curve. **Stroke work** (see Chapter 13) is often plotted instead of stroke volume as a useful indicator of function. The force of contraction is related to the degree of stretch of the muscle, and **Starling's Law of the Heart** is quoted as 'The energy released during contraction depends on the initial fibre length'.

The length–tension relationship

The relationship between cardiac muscle length and generation of force can be partly explained in terms of the **sliding filament theory** of muscle function. Briefly, as the muscle fibre is stretched, more crossbridges can form between myosin and actin (Fig. 14.1c), and force increases. The same process is seen in skeletal muscle, but in the heart an additional mechanism makes the relationship steeper. This probably involves a length-dependent increase in Ca^{2+} sensitivity of troponin-C (see Chapter 11).

Importance of Starling's Law

The most important consequence of Starling's Law is that the stroke volumes of the left and right ventricles are matched. Small transient differences in output occur all the time, e.g. during breathing or rising from a supine position, when CVP falls. However, if right ventricular output was greater than that from the left for any significant period, pulmonary blood volume and pressure would rise dramatically, and fluid would be forced into the lungs (**pulmonary oedema**). This does not normally happen because any increase in pulmonary blood pressure increases the filling pressure, and hence EDV, of the left ventricle. Left ventricular stroke volume then increases according to Starling's Law. Over a couple of beats it continues to increase until it has matched right ventricular output, so preventing any further rise in pulmonary venous pressure, and equilibrium is regained.

For the same reasons a rise in CVP will cause an increase in stroke volume from both right and left ventricles, that is an increase in cardiac output. Starling's Law will therefore also contribute to the rise in cardiac output during exercise when CVP may increase, and to the initial fall in cardiac output seen on standing, when CVP falls due to blood pooling in the legs. Starling's Law is an important compensatory mechanism in heart failure (see Chapter 43).

Effect of afterload

Another consequence of Starling's Law is that, within limits, stroke volume can be maintained in the face of an increase in blood pressure, or afterload. If blood pressure increases, the left ventricle has to pump against a higher load, and the amount of blood ejected is reduced. There is therefore more blood left in the ventricle at the end of systole (**end-systolic volume**, ESV). This, and the consequent rise in filling pressure due to the temporarily mismatched outputs (see above), contributes to refilling and EDV increases. As a result stroke volume and work

increases due to Starling's Law. Over the course of a few beats stroke volume therefore returns to its original value.

In summary, in the absence of any change in heart rate or cardiac muscle contractility, CVP is therefore the prime determinant of cardiac output (Fig. 14.1d).

Influence of the autonomic nervous system

The autonomic nervous system provides an external mechanism for regulating cardiac output, and is central to the control of blood pressure (see Chapters 26, 27). Sympathetic stimulation or application of epinephrine causes an increase in heart rate and contractile force, and the ventricular function curve is shifted upwards (Fig. 14.1b). A change in the ability of cardiac muscle to generate force *without any change in length* is called a change in **contractility**. Agents that alter contractility are known as **inotropic agents** or **inotropes**. Positive inotropes increase contractility, and include the sympathetic neurotransmitter norepinephrine. Negative inotropes decrease force, and include an increase in acidity. Note that the parasympathetic neurotransmitter acetylcholine is *not* a negative inotrope in the ventricles, and parasympathetic stimulation does not decrease contractility. The effects of the autonomic nervous system on heart rate and contractility, and inotropic and chronotropic agents, are discussed in more detail in Chapters 10 and 11.

Venous return and central venous pressure

Venous return, the volume of blood returning to the heart, must by definition equal cardiac output, except during very temporary perturbations. Venous return cannot 'control' cardiac output, except in so far as transient differences between cardiac output and venous return will alter CVP.

However, an increase in CVP will reduce the pressure gradient from the tissue capillaries to the heart, and therefore impede flow, i.e. venous return. If CVP were to rise sufficiently flow would cease. This would occur at the mean circulatory pressure (MCP, Fig. 14.1e), which is dependent on blood volume. During the steady state, cardiac output *must* equal venous return, so the apparently opposing effects of an increase in CVP on cardiac output (increase, Starling's Law) and venous return (decrease, pressure gradient) must reach an equilibrium. This is illustrated in Fig. 14.1e (*Guyton's analysis of flow*), where the effects of CVP on cardiac output and venous return are plotted together. The point at which the two lines cross is where the CVP results in equal cardiac output and venous return, and this will be the steady state.

As an example of how this works, in heart failure the ventricular function curve is depressed, but MCP is increased due to a greater blood volume as a result of venoconstriction and fluid retention. The new intersection point shows that cardiac output is almost returned to normal, but at the expense of a greatly increased CVP (Fig. 14.1e).

15 Electrical conduction system in the heart

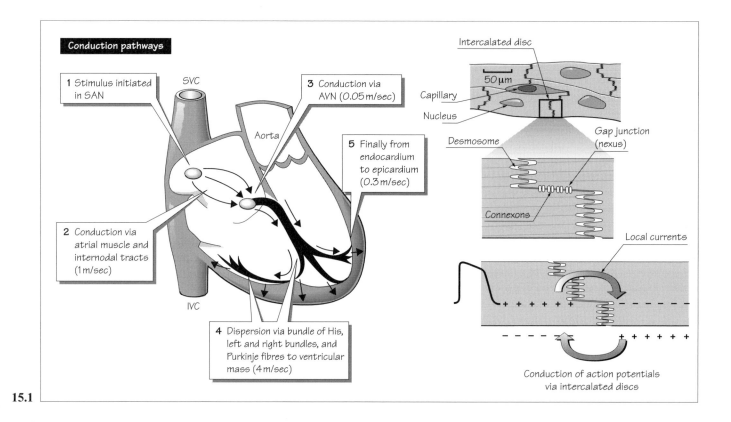

Conduction pathways

1 Stimulus initiated in SAN

SVC

3 Conduction via AVN (0.05 m/sec)

Aorta

5 Finally from endocardium to epicardium (0.3 m/sec)

2 Conduction via atrial muscle and internodal tracts (1 m/sec)

IVC

4 Dispersion via bundle of His, left and right bundles, and Purkinje fibres to ventricular mass (4 m/sec)

Intercalated disc

50 μm

Capillary

Nucleus

Desmosome

Gap junction (nexus)

Connexons

Local currents

+ + + + +

– – – – – – – + + + + + +

Conduction of action potentials via intercalated discs

15.1

Electrical conduction in cardiac muscle

Cardiac muscle cells are connected via **intercalated disks** (Chapter 2). These incorporate regions where the membranes of adjacent cells are very close, called **gap junctions**. Gap junctions consist of proteins known as **connexons**, which form low-resistance junctions between cells. They allow the transfer of small ions and thus electrical current. As all cells are therefore electrically connected, cardiac muscle is said to be a **functional** (or electrical) **syncytium**. If an action potential (AP) is initiated in one cell, local currents via gap junctions will cause adjacent cells to depolarize, initiating their own AP. A wave of depolarization will therefore be conducted from cell to cell throughout the myocardium. The rate of conduction is partly dependent on gap junction resistance and the *size of the depolarizing current*. This is related to the **upstroke velocity of the AP** (phase 0). Drugs that slow phase 0 slow conduction (e.g. lignocaine, class I antiarrhythmics). Pathological conditions such as ischaemia may increase gap junction resistance, and slow or abolish conduction. Retrograde conduction does not normally occur because the original cell is refractory (see Chapter 10). Transfer of the pacemaker signal from the sinoatrial node and synchronous contraction of the ventricles is facilitated by **conduction pathways** formed from modified muscle cells.

Conduction pathways in the heart
Sinoatrial node

The heart beat is normally initiated in the **sinoatrial node** (SAN), which is located at the junction of the superior vena cava and the right atrium. The SAN is a group of muscle cells that extends for ~2 cm down the sulcus terminalis and is ~2 mm wide. The cells are small and elongated, and have fewer striations than normal cardiac muscle cells. The SAN has a rich capillary supply and sympathetic and parasympathetic (right vagal) nerve endings. The SAN generates an AP about once a second (see Chapter 10).

Atrial conduction

The impulse spreads from the SAN across the right and left atria at ~1 m/s. Conduction to the **atrioventricular node** (AVN) is facilitated by larger cells in the three **internodal tracts** of Bachman (anterior), Wenckebach (middle), and Thorel (posterior).

The atrioventricular node

The atria and ventricles are separated by a nonconducting band, the **annulus fibrosus**. The AVN marks the upper region of the only conducting route through this band. The AVN is similar in structure to the SAN, and is situated near the interatrial septum and the mouth of the coronary sinus. It is innervated by sympathetic and left vagal nerves. The complex arrangement of small cells and slow AP upstroke (see Chapter 10) result in a very slow conduction velocity (~0.05 m/s). This provides a functionally significant delay of ~0.1 s between contraction of the atria and ventricles, which is reflected by the **P–R interval** of the **ECG**. Sympathetic stimulation increases conduction velocity and reduces the delay, whereas vagal stimulation slows conduction.

The bundle of His and Purkinje system

The bundle of His transfers the impulse from the AVN through the annulus fibrosus to the top of the interventricular septum. Close to the attachment of the septal cusp of the tricuspid valve it branches to form the **left and right bundle branches**. The left bundle divides further into the posterior and anterior fascicles. The bundles travel under the endocardium down the walls of the septum, and at the base divide into the multiple fibres of the **Purkinje system**. This distributes the impulse over the inner walls of the ventricles. Cells in the bundle of His and Purkinje system have a large diameter (~40 μm) and rapid AP upstroke velocity, and consequently a fast rate of conduction (~4 m/s). The impulse spreads from the Purkinje cells through the ventricular wall to the epicardium at 0.3–1 m/s, thereby initiating contraction.

Defects in conduction

Heart block

Complete **heart block (third degree)** occurs when conduction between atria and ventricles is abolished. This can result from ischaemic damage to nodal tissue or the bundle of His. In the absence of a signal from the SAN, the AVN and bundle of His can generate a heart rate of ~40 beats/min. Some Purkinje cells may also spontaneously generate APs, but at a rate of less than 20/min.

Abnormally slow conduction in the AVN can result in incomplete (**first-degree**) heart block, where the delay is much greater than normal, resulting in an extended P–R interval of the ECG. **Second-degree** heart block occurs when only a fraction of the impulses from the atria are conducted, so that, for example, ventricular contraction is only initiated every second or third atrial contraction (**2 : 1 or 3 : 1 block**). **Wenckebach block** (Mobitz I) is another type of second-degree block, in which the P–R interval progressively lengthens until there is no transmission from atria to ventricles and a QRS complex is missed; the cycle then begins again. Patients with first- or second-degree block are often asymptomatic (show no symptoms).

Bundle branch block

When one branch of the bundle of His does not conduct, the part of the ventricle that it serves will still be stimulated by conduction through the myocardium from unaffected areas. As this form of conduction is slower, activation is delayed and the QRS complex is broadened. This is called **left** or **right bundle branch block**.

Arrhythmias caused by congenital accessory conduction pathways

AV nodal re-entrant tachycardia (AVNRT) and **Wolff–Parkinson–White (WPW)** or **pre-excitation syndrome** are **arrhythmias** (disturbances of the cardiac rhythm) resulting in periodic episodes during which the heart rate abruptly increases to 150–250 beats per minute. Individuals with AVNRT have an additional (accessory) conduction pathway between the atrial muscle and the AVN. The normal AV pathway (termed α) conducts rapidly and has a long refractory period, while the accessory (β) pathway conducts slowly and has a short refractory period. In these individuals, AVNRT can be initiated when a *premature impulse* (see Chapter 45) is generated in the atrium. If the α pathway is still refractory from the preceeding impulse, it will not conduct the premature impulse. This impulse may, however, travel slowly down the β pathway (which has recovered from the preceeding impulse), and then encounter the distal end of the α pathway. Sufficient time has now elapsed for this pathway to be no longer refractory, and the impulse is able to ascend the α pathway in a retrograde direction, allowing it to return to the atrium. From here it can continue to cycle through the α and β pathways. This recycling of an impulse is known as **re-entry** or a **circus movement**. The ventricles are excited with each circuit, causing the tachycardia (increased heart rate).

WPW syndrome is an analogous condition in which the AVN is normal, but there is a separate congenital accessory conduction pathway (the **bundle of Kent**) between the atria and the ventricles. Impulses from the atrium are conducted to the ventricles via both the AVN and the bundle of Kent. The latter conducts more rapidly than the AVN so part of the ventricle is stimulated before the rest, resulting in a wide QRS complex (pre-excitation). Much like the α pathway in AVNRT, the bundle of Kent may have a long refractory period, and may not conduct premature impulses from the atrium. The AVN, however, is able to conduct these impulses, which reach the ventricles and can then return to the atrium via the bundle of Kent. The impulse can then set up a circus movement which encompasses the AVN, the His–Purkinje system, the ventricles, the bundle of Kent and an atrium.

16 The electrocardiogram

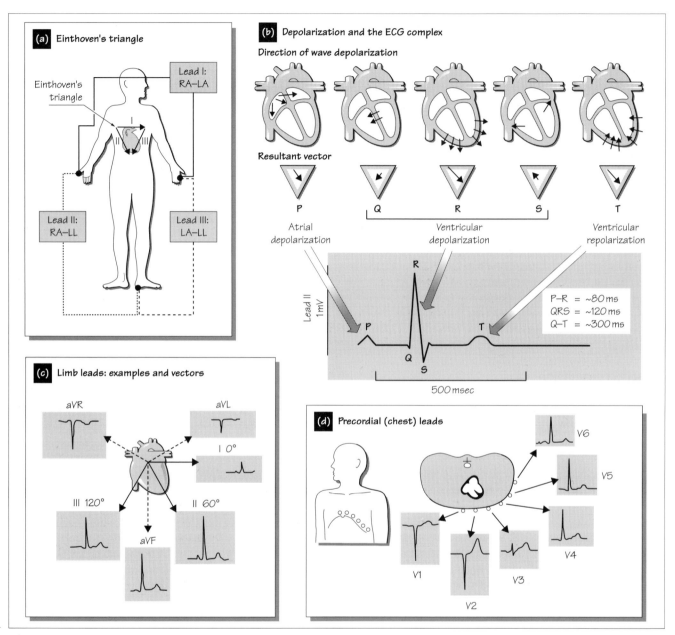

(a) Einthoven's triangle

Einthoven's triangle

Lead I:
RA–LA

Lead II:
RA–LL

Lead III:
LA–LL

(b) Depolarization and the ECG complex

Direction of wave depolarization

Resultant vector

P Q R S T

Atrial depolarization

Ventricular depolarization

Ventricular repolarization

Lead II 1mV

P–R = ~80 ms
QRS = ~120 ms
Q–T = ~300 ms

500 msec

(c) Limb leads: examples and vectors

aVR aVL

I 0°

III 120° II 60°

aVF

(d) Precordial (chest) leads

V6
V5
V4
V1
V3
V2

16.1

The extracellular fluids contain salts, and therefore conduct electricity. As these fluids are distributed throughout the body, the body acts as a **volume conductor**. When cardiac muscle depolarizes, extracellular currents between depolarized and resting cells cause potentials that can be measured at the body surface. These form the basis of the **electrocardiogram** (ECG).

Recording the ECG

The ECG is based around the concept of an equilateral triangle

(**Einthoven's triangle**), with the heart as the current source at its centre (Fig. 16.1a). The points of the triangle are approximated by the limb leads, connected to the right arm, left arm, and left leg. The potential difference between two leads will depend on the amplitude of the current, related to muscle mass, and the direction of current flow. There is a directional component because maximum potential occurs in line with the maximum current flowing between depolarized and resting tissue. The ECG thus has both amplitude and direction, and is a **vector quantity** (Fig. 16.1b).

By convention, the ECG is connected in such a way that a positive voltage causes an upward deflection, and the paper speed of the recorder is normally 25 or 50 mm/s. Note that the term **lead**, when used for the ECG, refers to a measurement made for a particular configuration, not to the wires connected to the patient.

The classical bipolar leads of the ECG approximate the potential difference across the sides of Einthoven's triangle, and are essentially looking at electrical activity in the heart from three different directions, separated by 60°. They are **Lead I**, measured as the potential difference between the right and left arm; **Lead II**, right arm and left leg; and **Lead III**, left leg and left arm. Lead II normally has the largest deflections, as it lies closest to the direction of ventricular depolarization. As the ventricles have the largest muscle mass, they give the largest current and thus voltage.

The unipolar leads use a single sensing electrode, and the voltage measured is the potential difference between this and an estimate of zero potential. Practically, the latter is obtained by connecting the limb leads together via a resistor. This approximates to the centre of the current source and hence Einthoven's triangle, i.e. the heart. Nine unipolar leads are commonly used clinically, consisting of six chest (**precordial**) leads, V1–V6, and the **augmented** leads aVR, aVL, and aVF. The chest leads use a separate sensing electrode placed on the chest (Fig. 16.1d), whereas the augmented leads use a limb lead as a sensing electrode (right arm, aVR; left arm, aVL; left leg, aVF), with the remaining two limb leads connected together to give the zero potential estimate. As the augmented leads measure between one point of Einthoven's triangle and the centre, they are seeing the heart at an angle rotated by 30° compared to the bipolar leads. The six limb leads together therefore give a view of the electrical activity of the heart every 30° (Fig. 16.1c).

General features of the ECG

The ECG trace has three main components that are related to the amplitude and direction of the wave of depolarization (vector) at that moment (Fig. 16.1b). The **P wave** is a small deflection due to depolarization of the atria. This is followed by the **QRS complex**, which is generally ~0.08 s in duration and reflects ventricular depolarization. It is the largest deflection because of the large ventricular muscle mass. It obscures the much smaller deflection related to repolarization of the atria. The relative size of the Q, R and S components varies between leads, and is dependent on the orientation of the heart. In lead II the Q wave is seen as a small downward deflection, correlating to the left to right depolarization of the interventricular septum. The R wave is a strong upwards deflection, corresponding to depolarization of the main mass of the ventricles. The S wave is a small downward deflection in lead II, and relates to depolarization of the last part of the ventricles close to the base of the heart. The **T wave**

corresponds to ventricular repolarization. As the mass of the conducting system (sinoatrial and atrioventricular node, bundle of His) is very small, the associated currents are too small to cause any appreciable deflection in the ECG.

The **P–R** and **S–T segments** are normally **isoelectric**, i.e. at zero potential. There is no potential because no current is flowing; the relevant tissue (atria or ventricles) is either all depolarized or all at rest. The nonconducting *annulus fibrosus* prevents current flow between the atria and ventricles during the P–R segment. The **P–R interval** reflects the delay between atrial and ventricular depolarization, and is largely related to the delay in the atrioventricular node. It is measured from the beginning of the P wave to the beginning of the QRS complex, and ranges from 0.12 to 0.20 s. It shortens as heart rate increases.

The **S–T segment** approximates to the plateau of the ventricular muscle action potential (AP), and is ~0.35 s. When the myocardium is injured, e.g. during ischaemia, some cells will be partially depolarized causing **injury currents** between them and undamaged tissue. This can either depress or elevate the ECG baseline. However, during the S–T segment all cells are completely depolarized. This gives rise to an apparent elevation or depression of the S–T segment, although it is actually the baseline that has altered. This is a common indication for acute myocardial damage such as a **myocardial infarction**.

Why the T wave is positive: The QRS complex in lead II is positive because the wave of depolarization progresses from the apex of the heart towards the base. As the T wave reflects repolarization it might be expected to be negative, because polarity is reversed. However, the length of the AP at the apex is longer than that at the base. Therefore although the apex depolarizes first, it repolarizes last, and the wave of repolarization progresses from the base towards the apex. The change in both polarity and direction cancel out, and the T wave is upwards. In pathological conditions where the AP is prolonged, or conduction from apex to base is slow, repolarization at the base may be delayed until after that at the apex. Under these conditions the T wave will be *inverted*.

The electrical axis of the heart

The angle of the ECG vector at its maximum amplitude is called the electrical axis of the heart. It corresponds to the point of maximum current developed during the heart beat, and hence depolarization of the main mass of the ventricles. It can be calculated from the three bipolar leads, which are at 60° to each other, and normally lies closest to lead II. Changes in the position of the heart will alter the axis, e.g. during breathing. An increase in mass of one of the ventricles will shift the axis in that direction. Thus left ventricular hypertrophy will cause **left axis deviation**, and right ventricular hypertrophy **right axis deviation**.

17 Haemodynamics

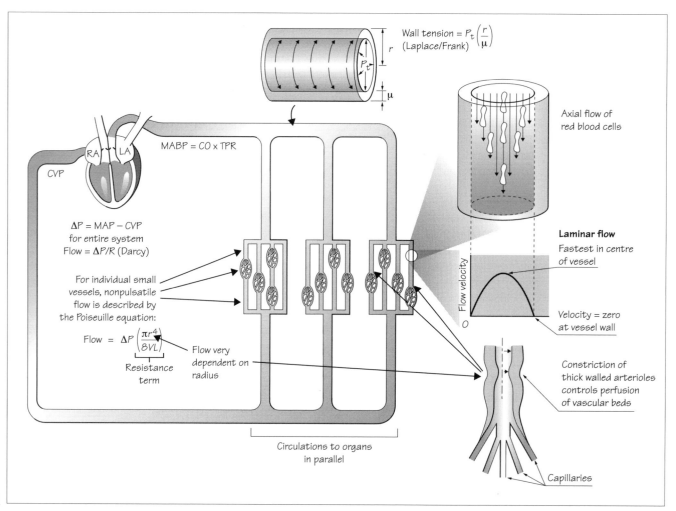

Wall tension = $P_t\left(\dfrac{r}{\mu}\right)$
(Laplace/Frank)

$MABP = CO \times TPR$

CVP

$\Delta P = MAP - CVP$
for entire system
Flow = $\Delta P/R$ (Darcy)

For individual small
vessels, nonpulsatile
flow is described by
the Poiseuille equation:

Flow = $\Delta P\left(\dfrac{\pi r^4}{8VL}\right)$

Resistance
term

Flow very
dependent on
radius

Circulations to organs
in parallel

Axial flow of
red blood cells

Laminar flow
Fastest in centre
of vessel

Velocity = zero
at vessel wall

Constriction of
thick walled arterioles
controls perfusion
of vascular beds

Capillaries

17.1

Relationships between pressure, resistance, and flow

Haemodynamics is the study of the relationships between **pressure**, **resistance** and the **flow of blood** in the cardiovascular system. Although the properties of this flow are enormously complex, they can largely be derived from simpler physical laws governing the flow of liquids through single tubes.

When a fluid is pumped through a system, its flow (Q) is determined by the pressure head developed by the pump ($P_1 - P_2$ or ΔP), and by the resistance (R) to that flow, according to **Darcy's law** (analogous to Ohm's law):

$$Q = \Delta P/R$$

or for the cardiovascular system as a whole:

$$CO = (MABP - CVP)/TPR$$

Where CO is cardiac output, $MABP$ is mean arterial blood pressure, TPR is total peripheral resistance and CVP is central venous pressure. Since CVP is ordinarily close to zero, $MABP$ is equal to $CO \times TPR$.

Resistance to flow is caused by frictional forces within the fluid, and depends on the viscosity of the fluid and the dimensions of the tube, as described by **Poiseuille's law**:

$$resistance = 8VL/\pi r^4$$

so that:

$$flow = \Delta P\pi r^4/8VL$$

Here, V is the viscosity of the fluid, L is the tube length, and r is the inner radius (= 1/2 the diameter) of the tube. Because flow depends on the 4th power of the tube radius in this equation, *small changes in radius have a powerful effect on flow*. For example, a 20% decrease in radius reduces flow by about 60%.

Considering the cardiovascular system as a whole, the different types or sizes of blood vessels (e.g. arteries, arterioles,

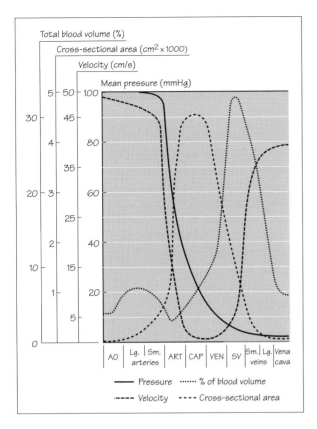

Total blood volume (%)
Cross-sectional area (cm² x 1000)
Velocity (cm/s)
Mean pressure (mmHg)

| AO | Lg. arteries | Sm. arteries | ART | CAP | VEN | SV | Sm. veins | Lg. veins | Vena cava |

—— Pressure ⋯⋯ % of blood volume
- - - - Velocity - - - Cross-sectional area

17.2

capillaries) are arranged sequentially, or in **series**. In this case, the resistance of the entire system is equal to the *sum of all the resistances* offered by each type of vessel:

$$R_{total} = R_{arteries} + R_{arterioles} + R_{capillaries} + R_{venules} + R_{veins}$$

Calculations taking into account the estimated lengths, radii and numbers of the various sizes of blood vessels show that the arterioles, and to a lesser extent the capillaries and venules, are primarily responsible for the resistance of the cardiovascular system to the flow of blood. In other words, $R_{arteriole}$ makes the largest contribution to R_{total}. Because according to Darcy's law the pressure drop in any section of the system is proportional to the resistance of that section, the steepest fall in pressure is in the arterioles (see Fig. 17.2).

Although the various sizes of blood vessel are arranged in series, each organ or region of the body is supplied by its own major arteries that emerge from the aorta. The vascular beds for the various organs are therefore arranged in **parallel** with each other. Similarly, the vascular beds within each organ are mainly arranged into parallel subdivisions (e.g. the arteriolar resistances $R_{arteriole}$ are in parallel with each other). For 'n' vascular beds arranged in parallel:

$$1/R_{total} = 1/R_1 + 1/R^2 + 1/R_3 + 1/R_4 \ldots 1/R_n$$

An important consequence of this relationship is that the bloodflow to a particular organ can be altered (by adjustments of the resistances of the arterioles in that organ) without greatly affecting pressures and flows in the rest of the system. This can

be accomplished, as a consequence of Poiseuille's law, by relatively small dilatations or constrictions of the arterioles within an organ or vascular bed.

Because there are so many small blood vessels (e.g. millions of arterioles, billions of venules, trillions of capillaries), the overall cross-sectional area of the vasculature reaches its peak in the microcirculation. As the velocity of the blood at any level in the system is equal to the total flow (the cardiac output) divided by the cross-sectional area at that level, the blood flow is slowest in the capillaries (see Fig. 17.2), favouring O_2/CO_2 exchange and tissue absorption of nutrients. The capillary transit time at rest is 0.5–2 s.

Blood viscosity

Very viscous fluids like motor oil flow more slowly than less viscous fluids like water. **Viscosity** is caused by frictional forces within a fluid which resist flow. Although the viscosity of plasma is similar to that of water, the viscosity of blood is normally three to four times that of water, because of the presence of blood cells, mainly erythrocytes. In **anaemia**, where the cell concentration (haematocrit) is low, viscosity and therefore vascular resistance decrease, and CO rises. Conversely, in the high-haematocrit condition **polycythaemia**, vascular resistance and blood pressure are increased.

Laminar flow

As liquid flows steadily through a long tube, frictional forces are exerted by the tube wall. These, in addition to viscous forces within the liquid, set up a *velocity gradient* across the tube (see Fig. 17.1) in which the fluid adjacent to the wall is motionless, and the flow velocity is greatest at the centre of the tube. This is termed **laminar flow**, and occurs in the microcirculation, except in the smallest capillaries. One consequence of laminar flow is that erythrocytes tend to move away from the vessel wall and align themselves edgewise in the flow stream. This reduces the effective viscosity of the blood in the microcirculation (the **Fåhraeus–Lindqvist effect**), helping to minimize resistance.

Wall tension

In addition to the pressure gradient along the length of blood vessels, there exists a pressure difference across the wall of a blood vessel. This *transmural pressure* is equal to the pressure inside the vessel minus the interstitial pressure. The transmural pressure exerts a circumferential *tension* on the wall of the blood vessel that tends to distend it, much as high pressure within a balloon stretches it. According to the **Laplace/Frank law**:

$$\text{wall tension} = P_t r/\mu$$

where P_t is the transmural pressure, r is the vessel radius, and μ is the wall thickness. In the aorta, where P_t and r are high, atherosclerosis may cause thinning of the arterial wall, and the development of a bulge or **aneurysm** (Chapter 32). This increases r and decreases μ, setting up a vicious cycle of increasing wall tension which, if not treated, may result in vessel rupture.

Blood pressure and flow in the arteries and arterioles

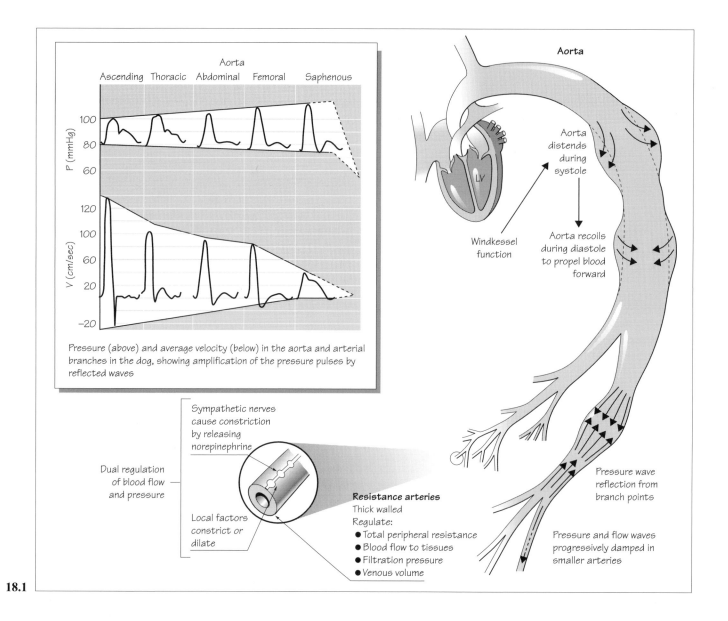

Pressure (above) and average velocity (below) in the aorta and arterial branches in the dog, showing amplification of the pressure pulses by reflected waves

18.1

Factors controlling arterial blood pressure

The mean arterial blood pressure is equal to the product of the cardiac output (about 5 L/min at rest) and the total peripheral resistance (TPR). Since the total drop of mean pressure across the systemic circulation is about 100 mmHg, TPR is calculated to be 100 mmHg/5000 ml/min, or 0.02 mmHg/ml/min. The unit mmHg/ml/min is referred to as a peripheral resistance unit (PRU), so that TPR is normally about 0.02 PRU.

Systolic pressure is mainly influenced by the stroke volume, the left ventricular ejection velocity, and aortic/arterial stiffness, and rises when any of these increase. Conversely, diastolic pressure rises with an increase in TPR. Arterial pressure falls progressively during diastole (see Fig. 13.1), so that a shortening of the diastolic interval associated with a rise in the heart rate also increases diastolic pressure.

Blood pressure and flow in the arteries

The bloodflow in the aorta and the larger arteries is *pulsatile*, as a result of the rhythmic emptying of the left ventricle.

As blood is ejected from the left ventricle during systole, it hits the column of blood already present in the ascending aorta, creating a *pressure wave* in the aortic blood which is rapidly (at between 4 and 10 m/s) conducted towards the arterioles. As this pulse pressure wave passes each point along the aorta and the major arteries, it sets up a transient pressure gradient that briefly propels the blood at that point forward, causing a pulsatile *flow*

	Vasoconstrictors	Vasodilators
Neurotransmitters	Sympathetic Norepinephrine ATP Neuropeptide Y	Parasympathetic and sensory (limited distribution) Acetylcholine (acts via NO) Substance P Calcitonin gene-related peptide Vasoactive intestinal peptide
Hormones	Epinephrine (most blood vessels) Vasopressin (antidiuretic hormone)	Epinephine (in skeletal muscle, coronary, hepatic arteries) Atrial natriuretic peptide
Endothelium-derived substances	Endothelin Endothelium-derived constricting Factor (chemical identity unknown)	Endothelium-derived relaxing factor (NO) Prostaglandin I_2 (prostacyclin) Endothelium-derived hyperpolarizing factor (chemical identity unknown)
Metabolites and related factors	Hypoxia (pulmonary arteries only)	Hypoxia (other vessels) Adenosine, hyperosmolarity, H^+ ions, lactic acid, K^+ ions, CO_2
Other locally produced factors	Histamine (veins, pulmonary arteries) Prostaglandin $F_{2\alpha}$, thromboxane A_2 5-Hydroxytryptamine Growth factors (e.g. PDGF)	Histamine (arterioles) Prostaglandin E_2 Bradykinin
Other factors	Pressure (myogenic response) Moderate cold (skin)	Increased flow Heat (skin)

wave. The blood in the arteries therefore moves forward in short bursts, separated by longer periods of stasis, so that its average velocity in the aorta is about 0.2 m/s.

The pressure wave also causes the elastic arterial wall to bulge out, thereby storing some of the energy of the wave. The arterial wall then rebounds, releasing part of this energy to drive the blood forward during diastole (*diastolic runoff*). This pumping mechanism of the elastic arteries is termed the **Windkessel** function (Fig. 18.1).

The large arteries also absorb and dissipate some of the energy of the pressure wave. This progressively damps the oscillations in flow, as shown by the lower traces in the inset to Fig. 18.1. However, as the upper traces illustrate, the pulse pressure wave becomes somewhat *larger* as it moves down the aorta and major arteries (e.g. the saphenous artery), before it then progressively dies out along the smaller arteries. This occurs in part because a fraction of the pressure wave is *reflected* back towards the heart at arterial branch points. In the aorta and large arteries, the reflected wave *summates* with the forward-moving pulse pressure wave, increasing its amplitude. Once the blood has entered the smaller arteries, however, the damping properties of the arterial wall predominate, and progressively depress the oscillations in flow and pressure, so that these die out completely by the time the blood reaches the microcirculation.

Arterioles and vascular resistance

The mean blood pressure falls progressively along the arterial system. The decline is particularly steep in the smallest arteries and the arterioles (diameter < 100 μm), because these vessels present the greatest resistance to flow (Fig. 17.2). The walls of the arterioles are very thick in relation to the diameter of the lumen, and these vessels can therefore constrict powerfully, dramatically increasing this resistance. Because the arterioles are normally partially constricted, their resistance can also be decreased by vasodilatatory stimuli.

The role of the arterioles in setting the vascular resistance has several important implications:

1 Constriction or dilatation of all, or a large proportion, of the arterioles in the body will affect the TPR and the blood pressure.

2 Constriction of the arterioles in one organ or region will selectively direct the flow of blood away from that region, while dilatation will have the opposite effect.

3 Changes in arteriolar resistance in a region affect the 'downstream' hydrostatic pressure within the capillary beds and veins in that region. Changes in the pressure within the capillaries affect the movement of fluid from the blood to the tissues (see Chapter 20). Because the veins are very compliant, their volume is very sensitive to alterations in pressure (see Chapter 21). Thus, arteriolar constriction in a region of the body will both promote the movement of fluid from its tissue spaces into its exchange vessels, and also decrease its venous volume. Both effects work to increase the blood supply to other parts of the body.

The table lists important endogenous substances and factors which affect arteriolar tone.

19 The microcirculation and the lymphatic system

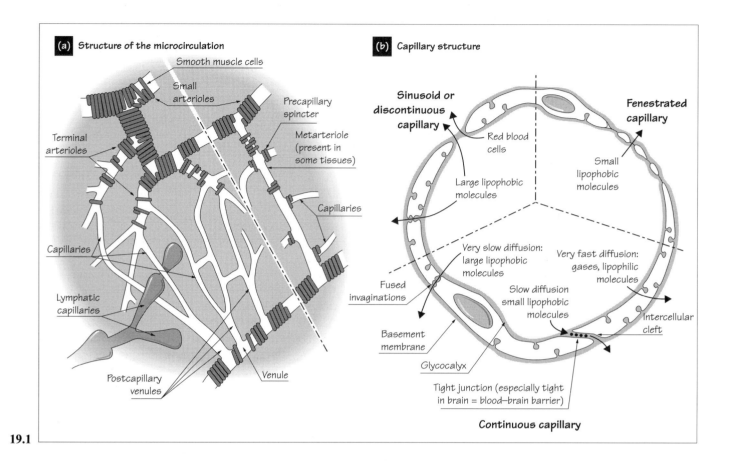

(a) Structure of the microcirculation

(b) Capillary structure

19.1

The **microcirculation** comprises the **smallest arterioles**, and the **exchange vessels**, including the **capillaries** and the **postcapillary venules**. The transfer of gases, water, nutrients, waste materials and other substances between the blood and body tissues carried out by the exchange vessels is the ultimate function of the cardiovascular system.

Organization of the microcirculation

Blood enters the microcirculation via small arterioles, the walls of which contain smooth muscle cells. These vessels are densely innervated by the sympathetic system, particularly in the splanchnic and cutaneous vascular beds. Sympathetically mediated constriction of each small arteriole reduces the blood-flow to many capillaries.

In some tissues (e.g. mesentery) capillaries branch from **thoroughfare vessels** which run from small arterioles to venules (Fig. 19.1a, right). The proximal (arteriolar) end of such a vessel is termed a **metarteriole**, and it is wrapped intermittently in smooth muscle cells. The capillaries have a ring of smooth muscle called a **precapillary sphincter** at their origin, but thereafter lack smooth muscle cells. Constriction of the precapillary sphincter controls the flow of blood through that capillary.

Most tissues, however, lack metarterioles or precapillary sphincters *per se*. Instead, the smallest or **terminal** arterioles divide to give rise to sets of capillaries (Fig. 19.1a, left). The terminal arteriole itself acts as a functional precapillary sphincter for its entire cluster of capillaries. Terminal arterioles are not innervated, and their tone is controlled by local metabolic factors (see Chapter 22). Under basal conditions, terminal arterioles constrict and relax periodically. This **vasomotion** causes the flow of blood through the cluster of capillaries to fluctuate.

The capillaries join to form *postcapillary venules*, which also lack smooth muscle cells. These merge to form *venules*, which contain smooth muscle cells and are sympathetically innervated.

Movement of solutes across the capillary wall

Water, gases and solutes (e.g. electrolytes, glucose, proteins) cross the walls of exchange vessels mainly by **diffusion**, a passive process by which substances move down their concentration gradients. O_2 and CO_2 can diffuse through the lipid bilayers of the endothelial cells. These and other **lipophilic** substances (e.g. general anaesthetics) therefore cross the capillary wall very rapidly. However, the lipid bilayer is impermeable to electrolytes and small **hydrophilic** (lipid-insoluble) molecules such as glucose, which therefore cross the walls of **continuous** capillaries (Fig. 19.1b, bottom) 1000–10 000 times more slowly than does O_2. Hydrophilic molecules cross the capillary wall mainly by diffusing between the endothelial cells. This process is slowed by *tight junctions* between the endothelial cells which impede diffusion through the intercellular clefts. Diffusion is also retarded by the **glycocalyx** and **basal lamina** —dense networks of fibrous macromolecules coating the luminal and abluminal sides of the endothelium, respectively. This tortuous diffusion pathway (the **small pore** system) acts as a sieve which admits molecules of molecular weight less than 10 000.

Even large proteins (e.g. albumin, MW 69 000) can cross the capillary wall, albeit very slowly. This suggests that the capillary wall also contains a small number of **large pores**, although these have never been directly visualized. It has been proposed that large pores exist transiently when membrane invaginations on either side of the endothelial cell fuse, temporarily creating a channel through which large molecules diffuse.

The endothelial cells of **fenestrated** capillaries (found in kidneys, intestines, and joints) contain pores called **fenestrae** (Fig. 19.1b, upper right). Fenestrated capillaries are about 10 times more permeable than are continuous capillaries to small hydrophilic molecules, because these can move through the fenestrae. **Sinusoidal** or **discontinuous** capillaries (liver, bone marrow, spleen) are very highly permeable, because they have wide spaces between adjacent endothelial cells through which proteins and even erythrocytes can pass (Fig. 19.1b, upper left).

The blood–brain barrier

The composition of the extracellular fluid in the brain must be kept extremely constant in order to allow stable neuronal function. This is made possible by the existence of the **blood–brain barrier** (BBB), which tightly controls the movement of ions and solutes across the walls of the continuous capillaries within the brain and the choroid plexus. The BBB has two important features. First, the junctions between the endothelial cells of cerebral capillaries are extremely tight (resembling the *zonae occludens* of epithelia), preventing any significant movement of hydrophilic solutes. Second, specialized membrane transporters exist in cerebral endothelial cells which allow the controlled movement of inorganic ions, glucose, amino acids and other substances across the capillary wall. Thus, the relatively uncontrolled diffusion of solutes present in other vascular beds is replaced in the brain by a number of specific transport processes. This can present a therapeutic problem, as most drugs are excluded from the brain (e.g. many antibiotics).

The BBB is interrupted in the **circumventricular organs**, areas of the brain which need to be influenced by blood-borne factors, or to release substances into the blood. These include the *pituitary* and *pineal* glands, the *median eminence*, the *area postrema*, and the *choroid plexus*. The BBB can break down with large elevations of blood pressure, osmolarity, or P_{CO_2}, and in infected areas of the brain.

The lymphatic system

Approximately 8 L of fluid containing solutes and plasma proteins is filtered from the microcirculation into the tissue spaces each day. This returns to the blood via the **lymphatic system**. Most body tissues contain *lymphatic capillaries* (Fig. 19.1a). These are blind-ended bulbous tubes 15–75 μm in diameter, with walls formed of a monolayer of endothelial cells. Interstitial fluid, plasma proteins and bacteria can easily enter the lymphatic capillaries via the gaps between these cells, the arrangement of which then prevents these substances from escaping. These vessels merge to form *collecting lymphatics*, the walls of which contain smooth muscle cells and one-way valves (as do the larger lymphatic vessels). The sections between these valves constrict strongly, forcing the lymph towards the blood. Lymph is also propelled by compression of the vessels by muscular contraction, body movement, and tissue compression. Lymph then enters the larger *afferent lymphatics*, which flow into the **lymph nodes**. Here, foreign particles and bacteria are scavenged by phagocytes, and can initiate immune reactions. Much of the lymph fluid is returned to the blood here via capillary absorption. The remaining fluid enters *efferent lymphatics*, most of which eventually merge into the *thoracic duct*. This duct empties into the left subclavian vein in the neck. Lymphatics from parts of the thorax, the right arm, and the right sides of the head and neck merge forming the *right lymph duct*, which enters the right subclavian vein. The lymphatic system is also important in the absorption of lipids from the intestines. The *lacteal* lymphatics are responsible for transporting about 60% of digested fat into the venous blood.

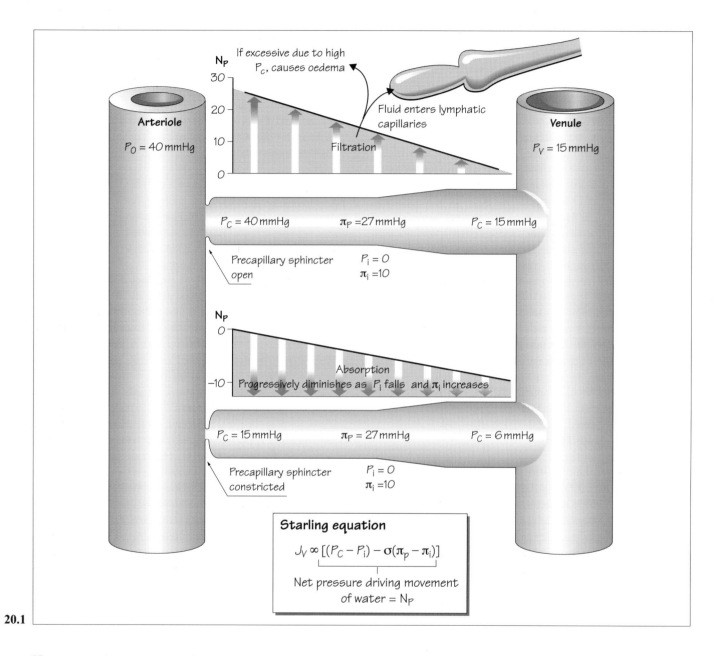

Starling equation

$$J_V \propto [(P_C - P_i) - \sigma(\pi_p - \pi_i)]$$

Net pressure driving movement of water = N_P

Movement of water across the capillary wall

The capillary wall (here taken to include also the wall of post-capillary venules) is very permeable to water molecules, which are able to pass easily in both directions through the plasma membranes of the endothelial cells. However, although individual water molecules can move freely between the plasma and the tissue spaces, the *net* flow of water across the capillary wall is quite small. This flow is determined by a balance between two forces or pressures which are exerted across the wall of the capillaries. These are a **hydrostatic pressure**, which tends to drive water out of the capillary, and an **osmotic pressure**, which tends

to draw water in from the surrounding tissue spaces. The sum of these two pressures at each point along the capillary is equal to a net pressure that will be directed either out of or into the capillary. The net flow of water is then proportional to this net pressure. The relationship between net flow (J_v) and the hydrostatic and osmotic pressures is described by the Starling equation:

$$J_v \propto [(P_c - P_i) - \sigma (\pi_p - \pi_i)]$$

The **hydrostatic force** ($P_c - P_i$) is equal to the difference between the blood pressure inside the capillary (P_c) and the pressure in the interstitium around the capillary (P_i). When capillaries are open (upper part of figure), P_c ranges from about 40 mmHg at the arteriolar end of the capillaries to about 15 mmHg in the venules. P_i is typically close to zero. The greater pressure inside the capillary tends to drive water out into the tissues.

As described in Chapter 19, the capillary wall acts as a *semipermeable membrane* or barrier to free diffusion, across which electrolytes and small molecules pass with much greater ease than plasma proteins. A substance dissolved on one side of a semipermeable membrane exerts an osmotic pressure that draws water across the membrane from the other side. This osmotic pressure is proportional to the concentration of the substance in solution, and is also a function of its permeability. Substances that can easily permeate a barrier (in this case the capillary wall) exert little osmotic pressure across it, whereas those which permeate less readily exert a larger osmotic pressure. For this reason, the osmotic force across the capillary wall is largely a result of the relatively impermeant plasma proteins, in particular albumin. The osmotic pressure exerted by plasma proteins is referred to as the **oncotic** or **colloid osmotic** pressure.

The osmotic force across the capillary wall is equal to the difference between the oncotic pressure of the plasma (π_p) and that of the interstitium (π_i), multiplied by a factor, the **reflection coefficient** (σ), which is a measure of how difficult it for the proteins to cross the capillary wall. Substances that cannot cross the membrane at all have a reflection coefficient of 1, while those that pass freely have a reflection coefficient of zero. σ ranges from about 0.8–0.95 for most plasma proteins, while ($\pi_p - \pi_i$) is typically about 17 mmHg.

Water filtration and absorption

Until recently, it was thought that the balance of forces described by the Starling equation was such that fluid tended to be *filtered* (i.e. to move out of the capillary) at the arteriolar end of the capillaries, and to be *absorbed* (move into the capillaries) at the venular end. However, the osmotic pressure term in the Starling equation is now thought to be somewhat smaller than previously estimated. Therefore, in most tissues, capillaries and venules that are being perfused with blood will be mainly filtering plasma (Fig. 20.1, upper part). On the other hand, certain sites such as the kidneys or the intestinal mucosa are specialized for water reabsorption. Here the osmotic pressure term is large, because plasma proteins are continually being washed out of the interstitium, so that net reabsorption occurs.

It is also the case that the balance between filtration and reabsorption is a dynamic one, mainly because the hydrostatic pressure within the capillaries is variable. Arteriolar vasodilatation, which increases intracapillary hydrostatic pressure, increases filtration, while arteriolar vasoconstriction favours absorption. For example, arterioles often demonstrate *vasomotion* (i.e. random opening and closing). During periods of arteriolar *constriction*, capillary pressure *falls*, favouring the *absorption* of interstitial fluid (Fig. 20.1, lower part). This absorption tends to be transient however, because as fluid moves into the capillaries P_i falls and π_i increases. Both effects progressively diminish absorption.

Assumption of the upright posture increases the transcapillary hydrostatic pressure gradient in the lower extremities, thereby immediately increasing filtration in these regions. However, this effect is partially compensated for by a rapid sympathetically mediated constriction of the arterioles in the legs, which reduces bloodflow and attenuates the rise in capillary hydrostatic pressure in these areas.

By the same token, fluid tends to accumulate in the tissue spaces of the upper body and face during the night, since assumption of the supine position increases capillary hydrostatic pressures above the heart. This causes morning 'puffiness'.

Normally, there is a slight predominance of filtration over absorption in the body as a whole. Of about 4000 L of plasma entering the capillaries daily as the blood recirculates, a *net* filtration of 8 L occurs. This fluid is returned to the vascular compartment through the lymphatic system.

Pulmonary and systemic oedema

The hydrostatic and osmotic pressures in the capillaries of the pulmonary circulation are atypical. Both P_c (7 mmHg) and P_i (−8 mmHg) are low, while π_i is high (14 mmHg), because these vessels are highly permeable to plasma proteins. The balance of forces slightly favours filtration. In **congestive heart failure**, the output of both the left and right ventricles is markedly reduced (Chapter 43). Failure of the left ventricle results in an increase in left ventricular end diastolic pressure. This pressure backs up into the lungs, causing increased pulmonary venular and capillary pressures. This promotes filtration in these vessels, causing an accumulation of fluid in the lungs (**pulmonary oedema**) which dramatically worsens the dysopnea (breathlessness) and inadequate tissue oxygenation characteristic of congestive heart failure. Similarly, failure of the right ventricle increases systemic venous and therefore capillary pressure, leading to systemic oedema, particularly of the lower extremities.

Oedema of the legs is also caused by **varicose veins**, a condition in which the venous valves are unable to operate properly because the veins become swollen and overstretched. By interfering with the effectiveness of the skeletal muscle pump, the incompetence of the valves leads to increases in venous and capillary hydrostatic pressure, resulting in the rapid development of oedema during standing.

21 The venous system

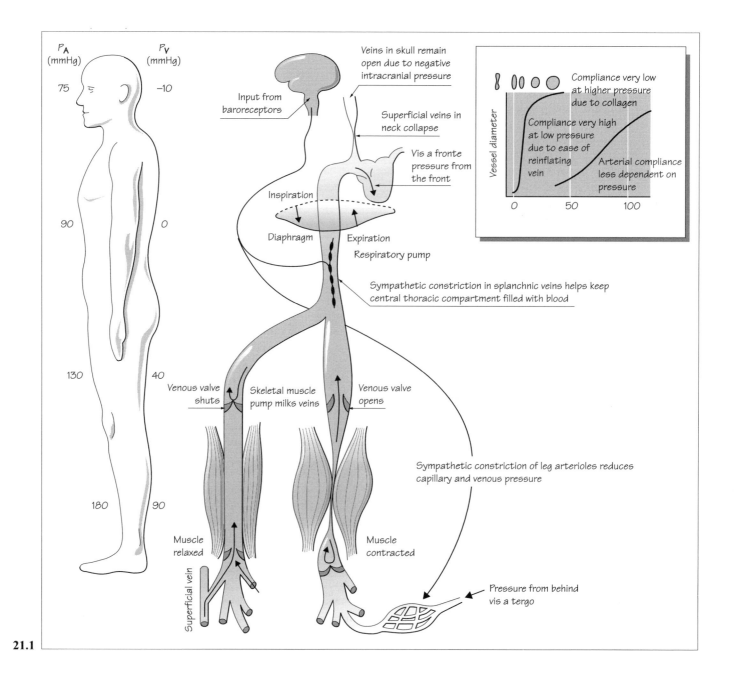

21.1

The venules and veins return the blood from the microcirculation to the right atrium of the heart. They do not, however, serve merely as passive conduits. Instead, they have a crucial active role in stabilizing and regulating the **venous return** of blood to the heart.

The venous system differs from the arterial system in two important respects. First, the total volume (and cross-sectional area) of the venous system is much greater than that of the arterial system. This is because there are many more venules than arterioles; venules also tend to have larger internal diameters than arterioles. Second, the veins are quite thin walled, and can therefore expand greatly to hold more blood if their internal pressure rises.

As a result of its large cross-sectional area, the venous system offers much less resistance to flow compared to the arterial system. The pressure gradient required to drive the blood through the venous system (15 mmHg) is therefore much smaller than the pressure needed in the arterial system (80 mmHg). The average pressure in the vena cavae (**the central venous pressure**) is usually close to 0 mmHg (i.e. atmospheric pressure). The flow of blood back to the heart is aided by the presence of one-way **venous valves** in the arms and especially the legs, which prevent backflow.

Venous arterial compliance

The graph in Fig. 21.1 (upper right) illustrates the relationship between pressure and volume in a typical vein and artery. The slope of the volume/pressure curve is referred to as **compliance**. Compliance is a measure of **expandability**. Veins are much more **compliant** than arteries at low pressures (0–10 mmHg). Small increases in venous pressure in this range therefore cause large increases in venous blood volume.

One reason for high venous compliance is that their thin walls allow veins to collapse at low internal pressures. Only small increases in pressure are needed to 'reinflate' a collapsed vein with blood until it has nearly rounded up. At higher pressures, however, venous compliance decreases dramatically (see graph) because the slack in rigid collagen fibres in the venous wall is rapidly taken up. This limit on the expandability of the veins is important in limiting the pooling of blood in the veins of the legs which occurs during standing.

The veins as capacitance vessels

Because of their large volumes and high compliance, the veins/venules accommodate a much larger volume of the blood (~70% of the total) than do the arteries/arterioles (~12%). They are therefore termed **capacitance vessels**, and are able to serve as *blood volume reservoirs*. During exercise, and in hypotensive states (e.g. during haemorrhage), sympathetically mediated constriction of the veins/venules, notably in the *splanchnic* (including the gastrointestinal tract and liver) and *cutaneous* circulations, displaces blood to other essential vascular beds, while also helping to maintain the blood pressure. At the same time, the resulting reduction of the venous volume increases the volume of blood in the *central thoracic compartment* (i.e. the heart and pulmonary circulation), thereby boosting cardiac output.

Effects of posture

When the upright position is assumed, the pull of gravity increases the absolute pressures within *both* the arteries and veins of the lower extremities. The average arterial and venous blood pressures in a normal adult standing quietly are about 100 and 0 mmHg at the level of the heart, while in the feet the pressures are about 190 and 90 mmHg, respectively. However, gravity does not affect the *pressure gradient* driving the blood circulation, because the *difference* between the arterial and venous pressures is similar (100 mmHg) at both levels. Standing therefore does not stop blood from flowing back to the heart.

The increased pressure within the veins of the lower extremities causes them to distend, so that about 500 ml of blood is immediately shifted into this part of the circulation. The rise in hydrostatic pressure within the capillaries of the lower extrem-ities increases fluid filtration, causing a progressive loss of plasma volume into the tissues of the legs and feet. The resulting loss of blood from the central thoracic compartment lowers stroke volume and cardiac output. As a result of these effects, cerebral bloodflow falls by 10–20%.

These potentially harmful effects are limited by the baroreceptor and cardiopulmonary reflexes, which respond to a fall in the pulse pressure (Chapter 26). These cause an *increased heart rate* and *vasoconstriction* in the lower extremities. This limits the loss of blood from the central thoracic compartment and slightly raises MAP and TPR. The cardiac output falls by about 20%. A local *sympathetic axon reflex* also reduces blood flow to the lower extremities, limiting fluid filtration.

In the upright position, the reduction of intravascular pressures above the heart causes the partial collapse of superficial veins, although the deeper veins remain partly open because their walls are anchored to surrounding tissues. Standing also causes a downward displacement into the spinal canal of the cerebrospinal fluid bathing the CNS, creating a negative pressure inside the rigid cranium that prevents cerebral veins from collapsing.

Several other mechanisms also aid venous return, particularly during exercise.

The skeletal muscle pump

Even during quiet standing, the leg muscles are stimulated by reflexes to contract and relax rhythmically, causing swaying. During contraction, veins within the muscles are squeezed, forcing blood towards the heart, as the venous valves prevent retrograde flow. Upon relaxation, these veins expand, drawing in blood from venules and from superficial veins that communicate with the muscle veins via collaterals (Fig. 21.1). This *skeletal muscle pump* thus 'milks' the veins, driving blood towards the heart and assisting venous return. The skeletal muscle pump is enormously potentiated during walking and running, causing a dramatic lowering of the venous pressure in the foot to levels as low as 30 mmHg.

The respiratory pump

During inspiration, the intrathoracic pressure falls and the intra-abdominal pressure rises, as a result of the downward displacement of the diaphragm. This increases the pressure gradient favouring venous return, and vena caval flow rises. An opposite effect occurs during expiration.

Effect of cardiac contraction

Downward displacement of the ventricles during systole pulls on the atria, expanding them and drawing in blood from the vena cavae and pulmonary veins. When the atrioventricular valves between the atria and ventricles then open during diastole, the blood is drawn in from these veins by the expansion of the ventricles, further aiding venous return. Venous return is therefore driven not only by the upstream pressure, but also (to a smaller extent) by downstream suction.

22 Local control of bloodflow

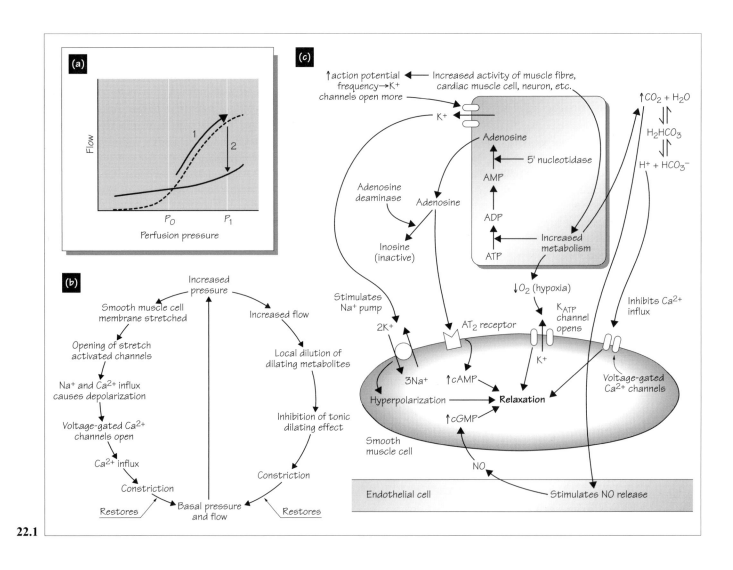

22.1

The activity of the sympathetic nervous system provides for centrally coordinated control of vascular tone (see Chapters 26, 27) and serves to maintain constant arterial blood pressure. There are, however, additional mechanisms that regulate vascular tone. Local mechanisms arise either from within the blood vessel itself, or from the surrounding tissue. These **local** mechanisms function primarily to regulate **flow**. Regulation tends to be most important in organs which require a constant blood supply, or in which metabolic needs may increase markedly (brain, kidneys, heart, skeletal muscles).

Local mechanisms have two main functions. First, under *basal conditions* they regulate local vascular resistance to maintain the bloodflow in many types of vascular beds at a nearly constant level over a large range of arterial pressures (50–170 mmHg). This tendency to maintain a *constant flow* during variations in pressure is termed **autoregulation**. Autoregulation prevents

major fluctuations in capillary pressure that would lead to uncontrolled movement of fluid into the tissues.

Second, when a tissue requires more blood to meet its metabolic needs, local mechanisms cause dilatation of resistance vessels and upregulate bloodflow. This response is referred to as **metabolic vasodilatation**. Autoregulation may persist under these conditions, but is adjusted to maintain flow around a higher or lower set point.

Autoregulation

Figure 22.1(a) illustrates the phenomenon of autoregulation. When the pressure driving blood through a resistance artery is suddenly increased to P_1 from its starting level P_0, the artery dilates passively and bloodflow immediately rises as predicted by Poiseuille's law (arrow 1). Within a minute, however, the resistance artery responds to the increased pressure by *actively constricting* (arrow 2), thereby bringing bloodflow back down towards its initial level (solid line). Similarly, decreases in pressure cause rapid compensatory dilatations to maintain flow. Autoregulation ensures that under basal conditions bloodflow remains nearly constant over a wide range of pressures, and is particularly important in the heart, the brain, and the kidneys. Two homeostatic negative feedback mechanisms are involved, the **myogenic response** and the effect of **vasodilating metabolites** (Fig. 22.1b).

The myogenic response is thought to be controlled mainly by sensors in the plasma membrane of smooth muscle cells, which react to changes in pressure and/or stretch. These include **stretch-activated channels**, which respond to increased pressure by opening to allow Na^+ and Ca^{2+} influx. The resulting cell depolarization opens voltage-gated Ca^{2+} channels, causing Ca^{2+} influx and vasoconstriction. The opposite process (i.e. hyperpolarization, closing of Ca^{2+} channels) occurs when pressure falls, causing vasodilatation.

Cellular metabolism results in the production of **vasodilating metabolites** or **factors** (Fig. 22.1c) which diffuse into the tissue spaces and affect neighbouring arterioles. If bloodflow increases, these substances tend to be washed out of the tissue, leading to an inhibition of vasodilatation that counteracts the rise in bloodflow. Conversely, decreased bloodflow causes a local accumulation of metabolites, leading to a homeostatic vasodilatation.

Metabolic and reactive hyperaemia

When metabolism in cardiac and skeletal muscle increases during exercise, tissue concentrations of vasodilating metabolites rise markedly. Similarly, focal changes in brain metabolism accompany diverse types of mental activity, causing enhanced local production of metabolites. The increased presence of such factors in the interstitium causes a powerful vasodilatation, termed **metabolic** or **functional hyperaemia**, allowing the rises in bloodflow necessary to supply the increased metabolic demand.

An accumulation of vasodilating metabolites also occurs during flow occlusion (e.g. caused by thrombosis). Release of occlusion then results in **reactive hyperaemia**; this is a large increase in bloodflow that hastens the re-establishment of cellular energy stores. This response is transient, persisting until levels of these metabolites fall back to normal levels.

Metabolic factors

Many factors contribute to metabolic vasodilatation. The most important factors are thought to be **adenosine**, **K^+ ions**, and **hypercapnia** (increased P_{CO_2}). Local **hypoxia** (reduced P_{O_2} deficit) can also relax vascular smooth muscle cells, partly by opening ATP-sensitive K^+ channels. **Inorganic phosphate**, **hyperosmolarity** and **lactic acid** may also act as metabolic dilators (not shown), although this is less well established.

Adenosine is a potent vasodilator that is released from the heart, skeletal muscles and brain during increased metabolism and hypoxia. It is thought to contribute to metabolic control of bloodflow in these organs. Adenosine is produced when AMP, which accumulates as a result of increased ATP breakdown, is dephosphorylated by the cell membrane enzyme **5'-nucleotidase**. It passes into the extracellular space, dilating neighbouring arterioles before being broken down to inosine by **adenosine deaminase**. It causes vasodilatation by acting on **A_2 receptors** to increase cAMP levels in vascular myocytes. It has other actions in the body (e.g. inhibiting conduction in the atrioventricular node). Some of these actions are mediated by **A_1 receptors** (which lower cAMP).

Ischaemia or increased activation of muscles and nerves causes K^+ ions to move out of cells. Resulting increases in the extracellular K^+ concentration (up to 10–15 mM) dilate arterioles, partly by stimulating the Na,K-ATPase, during functional hyperaemia in skeletal muscle and brain tissue. **Hypercapnia** associated with **acidosis** occurs in brain tissue during stimulation of local metabolism, and also during **cerebral ischaemia** (stroke). These are thought to provide a powerful vasodilating stimulus, both by releasing **nitric oxide** from endothelial cells, and by directly inhibiting Ca^{2+} influx into arteriolar cells.

Other local mechanisms

There are also a number of mechanisms acting locally in selected vascular beds under specific particular circumstances. For example, during the inflammatory reaction, local infection or trauma causes the release of various **autocoids** (local hormones), including the arteriolar dilators **histamine**, **prostaglandin E$_2$**, **bradykinin** and **platelet activating factor**. These increase local bloodflow and increase postcapillary venular permeability, thereby increasing the access of leucocytes and antibodies to damaged and infected tissues. The generation of **bradykinin** by sweat glands during sweating promotes cutaneous vasodilatation. **Prostaglandin I$_2$** (PGI$_2$, prostacyclin) is synthesized and released in the renal cortex under conditions where renal bloodflow is reduced by vasoconstrictors. Prostacyclin has a vasodilating action that helps to maintain renal bloodflow. Conversely, the release of **serotonin** (5-hydroxytryptamine) and **thromboxane A$_2$** from platelets during blood clotting causes vasospasm, which helps to reduce bleeding.

Regulation of the vasculature by the endothelium

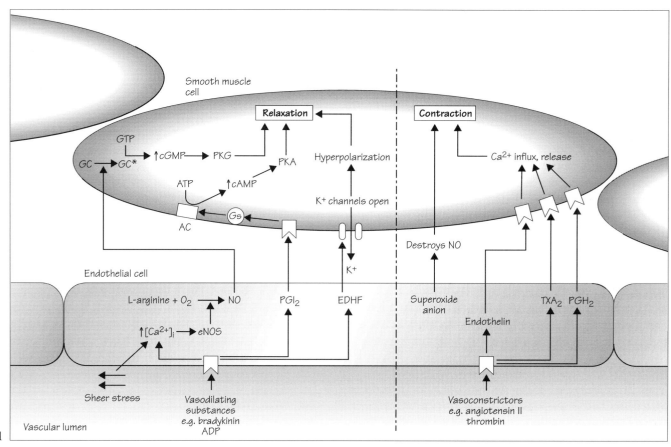

23.1

The inner surface of blood vessels is lined by a monolayer of endothelial cells and these are crucial in regulating vascular tone. When stimulated by substances present in the blood, or by the shear stress associated with the flow of blood, endothelial cells can release both constricting and dilating substances (Fig. 23.1). Important endothelial vasodilators include **endothelium-derived relaxing factor** (EDRF, now known to be **nitric oxide** or a closely related nitroso-containing compound), **prostacyclin** (PGI$_2$), and **endothelium-derived hyperpolarizing factor** (EDHF). The major endothelial vasoconstrictors are **endothelin-1, thromboxane A$_2$** (TXA$_2$), and **prostaglandin H$_2$**.

Endothelial cells also play a crucial role in suppressing platelet aggregation and thereby regulating haemostasis (see Chapter 7), and, as the major constituents of the capillary wall, control vascular permeability to many substances (Chapter 9).

Nitric oxide

Nitric oxide (chemical formula NO) is the most important vasodilator released by endothelial cells. NO is synthesized from the amino acid L-arginine and molecular oxygen by nitric oxide synthase (NOS). The most important form of NOS in the cardiovascular system is **endothelial NOS** (eNOS). This enzyme is responsible for a continual production and release of NO by endothelial cells (also by platelets and the heart). eNOS is activated when endothelial cell [Ca^{2+}]$_i$ is increased, leading to raised levels of the Ca^{2+}–calmodulin complex which stimulates the enzyme. Substances which cause vasodilatation in this way include locally released factors such as bradykinin, adenine, adenosine nucleotides, histamine, serotonin and the neurotransmitter substance P. Acetylcholine has a similar effect, although it is not known whether this has any physiological importance. There is also evidence that epinephrine and other β-adrenoceptor agonists cause NO release, possibly via a cyclic AMP-dependent mechanism that is independent of a rise in [Ca^{2+}]$_i$.

Once released from the endothelium, NO diffuses through the vascular wall and into the smooth muscle cells, where it activates the cytosolic enzyme **guanylyl cyclase**. This increases levels of cellular cyclic GMP, which causes relaxation by mechanisms described in Chapter 12. NO is quite reactive and is therefore broken down within several seconds, so that it has a strictly local effect.

Inducible NOS (iNOS) is expressed in macrophages, lymphocytes, vascular smooth muscle and many other types of cells during inflammation. iNOS is capable of producing much greater amounts of NO, and probably contributes to the destruction of foreign organisms by the immune system. An overproduction of NO by iNOS in septic shock is thought to contribute to the severe hypotension characterizing this condition.

The formation of NO can be competitively antagonized by L-arginine analogues such as L-nitro arginine methyl ester (L-NAME); these have proved to be useful experimental tools for evaluating the roles of NO *in vitro* and *in vivo*. It has been shown, for example, that infusion of L-NAME in humans causes a sustained rise in blood pressure and total peripheral resistance, suggesting that a tonic basal release of NO is acting to reduce the total peripheral resistance.

Pharmacological sources of NO

Organic nitrates such as **glyceryl trinitrate** and **isosorbide dinitrate** are acted on by the enzyme glutathione *S*-transferase in vascular smooth muscle to release nitrite ion (NO_2^-), which is then converted to NO to cause dilatation. These drugs, which dilate veins more effectively than arteries, are used to treat angina pectoris (see Chapter 39). The drug **sodium nitroprusside** releases NO spontaneously in both arterial and venous smooth muscle cells, and its powerful dilator effect on both arteries and veins is useful in the treatment of hypertensive emergencies and acute heart failure (see Chapter 44).

Other endothelium-derived relaxing factors

Prostacyclin is released from the endothelium by many of the factors that cause NO release. It promotes vasodilatation by increasing smooth muscle cell cyclic AMP levels, but its most important role is in limiting platelet attachment and aggregation. There is also extensive evidence that the endothelium releases a substance that contributes to relaxation by opening K+ channels in vascular smooth muscle cells, thereby causing hyperpolarization. The chemical nature of this factor, referred to as **endothelium-derived hyperpolarizing factor**, is unknown, as is its precise role *in vivo*.

Endothelium-derived constricting factors

Endothelin-1 is a peptide of 21 amino acids which is released by the endothelium in the presence of many vasoconstrictors, including angiotensin, vasopressin, thrombin, and epinephrine. Endothelin is a potent vasoconstricting agent, particularly in veins and arterioles, and stimulates two subtypes of receptor on vascular smooth muscle cells, designated ET_A and ET_B. Endothelin causes vasoconstriction via G-protein-linked mechanisms similar to those activated by norepinephrine. The infusion of endothelin receptor antagonists into humans causes a sustained fall in total peripheral resistance, implying that ongoing endothelin release contributes to maintaining the blood pressure.

Endothelial cells are also capable of releasing other vasoconstricting substances, including **prostanoids** (thromboxane A_2 and prostaglandin H_2) and superoxide anions, which may enhance constriction by breaking down NO. In addition, **angiotensin converting enzyme** (ACE) present on the surface of endothelial cells converts is responsible for the production of the vasoconstrictor angiotensin II (see Chapter 28), as well the breakdown of the potent vasodilator bradykinin.

The endothelium in cardiovascular disease

Many diseases that disturb vascular function are associated with abnormalities of the endothelium. Dysfunction of the endothelium is thought to contribute to the early stages of **atherosclerosis**, while damage to the endothelium is a crucial factor leading to thrombus formation in the advanced atherosclerotic lesion (see Chapter 34). Plasma from patients with **diabetes mellitus** contains abnormally high levels of biochemical markers indicative of endothelial damage, and there is evidence, both in animal models of insulin-dependent diabetes and in patients with this disorder, that endothelium-dependent relaxation is blunted. This deficit in endothelial function is thought to contribute to the increased risks of atherosclerosis, neuropathy and hypertension that are associated with diabetes. The mechanisms leading to diabetes-associated endothelial dysfunction remain incompletely defined, but may include damage by raised levels of glucose and/or oxidized low-density lipoproteins.

Endothelial dysfunction may also be important in causing **pre-eclampsia**, a disorder of pregnancy characterized by hypertension and increased blood clotting, which is the leading cause of maternal mortality. The endothelium is thought to play an important role in causing the fall in maternal blood pressure that normally occurs during pregnancy. This protective function may, however, be disrupted in patients suffering from pre-eclampsia, possibly due to the release of substances from the placenta which damage the endothelial cells.

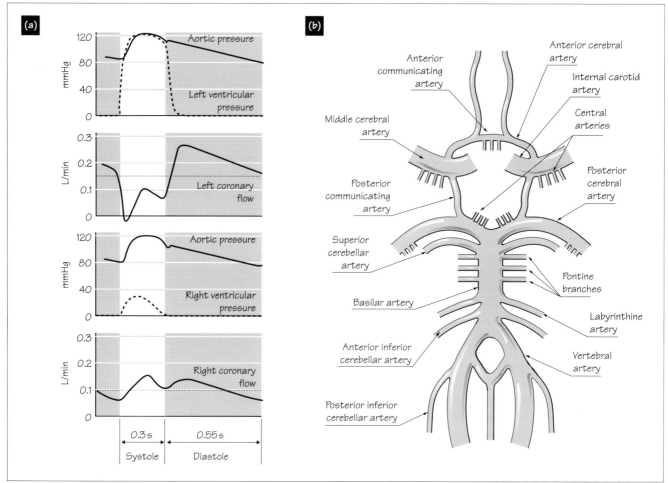

24.1

The vascular beds supplying the different organs of the body are structurally and functionally specialized, allowing an optimal matching of bloodflow with their individual requirements.

Coronary circulation

The **left** and **right coronary** arteries branch from the aorta just above the aortic valve. The left coronary artery gives rise to **left circumflex** and **anterior descending** branches which supply mainly the left ventricle and septum. The right coronary artery supplies mainly the right ventricle. Venous drainage of the heart occurs mainly (95%) into the right atrium via the **coronary sinus** and **anterior cardiac vein**. A small amount of venous blood also enters all cardiac chambers through **thebesian** and **anterior coronary** veins.

The *high capillary density* of the myocardium (~1 capillary per muscle cell), allows it to extract an unusually large fraction (about 70%) of the oxygen from its blood supply. The resting bloodflow to the heart is relatively high, and moreover increases approximately fivefold during strenuous exercise.

Figure 24.1(a) shows left and right coronary bloodflow during the cardiac cycle at a resting heart rate of 70 beats/min. During systole, the branches of the left coronary artery which penetrate the myocardial wall to supply the subendocardium of the left ventricle are strongly compressed by the high pressure within the ventricle and its wall. Left coronary bloodflow is therefore almost abolished during systole, so that 85% of flow occurs during diastole. Conversely, right coronary arterial flow rate is highest during systole, because the aortic pressure driving flow increases more during systole (from 80 to 120 mmHg) than the right ventricular pressure which opposes flow (from 0 to 25 mmHg).

With a heart rate of 70 beats/min, systole and diastole last 0.3 and 0.55 s, respectively. As the heart rate increases during exercise or excitement, however, the duration of diastole shortens more than that of systole. At 200 beats/min, for example, systole and diastole both last for 0.15 s. In order to cope with the greatly increased oxygen demand of the heart, which occurs simultaneously with a marked reduction in the time available for left coronary perfusion, the coronary arteries/arterioles dilate dramatically to allow for a pronounced rise in bloodflow. Dilatation is caused by *vasodilating factors*, including **adenosine**, **hypoxia**, and **K+**, which are generated as a result of *increased cardiac metabolism. The heart therefore regulates its own blood supply via a well-developed* **metabolic hyperaemia** (see Chapter 22).

Skeletal muscle circulation

The skeletal muscles comprise about 50% of body weight, and at rest receive 15–20% of cardiac output. At rest, skeletal muscle arterioles have a high basal tone as a result of tonic sympathetic vasoconstriction. At any one time, most muscle capillaries are not perfused, due to intermittent constriction of precapillary sphincters (vasomotion).

Because the muscles form such a large tissue mass, their arterioles make a major contribution to total peripheral resistance. Sympathetically mediated alterations in their arteriolar tone therefore play a crucial role in regulating total peripheral resistance and blood pressure during operation of the baroreceptor reflex. The muscles thus serve as a '*pressure valve*' that can be closed to increase blood pressure and opened to lower it.

With *rhythmic exercise*, compression of blood vessels during the contraction phase causes the bloodflow to become intermittent. However, increased muscle metabolism causes the generation of *vasodilating factors*; these factors cause an enormous increase in bloodflow during the relaxation phase, especially to the white or *phasic* fibres involved in movement. With maximal exercise, the skeletal muscles receive 80–90% of cardiac output. Vasodilating factors include **K+ ions**, **CO2**, and **hyperosmolarity**. In working muscle their effects completely *override* sympathetic vasoconstriction, while arterioles in nonworking muscle remain sympathetically constricted so that their bloodflow does not increase.

Sustained compression of blood vessels during *static* (isometric) muscle contractions causes an occlusion of flow that rapidly results in muscle fatigue.

Cutaneous circulation

Apart from supplying the relatively modest metabolic requirements of the skin, the main function of the cutaneous vasculature is to maintain a constant body temperature. **Thermoregulation** is aided by the presence of **arteriovenous anastomoses** (AVA). AVA are coiled, thick-walled thoroughfare blood vessels, which connect arterioles and veins directly, bypassing the capillaries. AVA are located mainly in the skin of the *hands, feet, lips, nose*, and *ears*. When open, AVA allow a high-volume bloodflow into a cutaneous venous *plexus* (network) from which heat can be radiated to the environment.

The sympathetic nervous system acts through α_1-*receptors* to control the resistance of AVAs and also cutaneous arterioles and veins. A fall in temperature, sensed by peripheral and hypo-thalamic thermoreceptors, causes a hypothalamically mediated increase in sympathetic outflow to the skin. This causes the AVAs and cutaneous arterioles and veins to constrict. This minimizes the loss of body heat by producing a pronounced decrease in cutaneous bloodfow, which can fall to one-tenth of its thermoneutral level of 10–20 ml/min/100 g.

With an increased temperature, decreased sympathetic outflow allows the AVAs and other cutaneous blood vessels to open, bringing blood to the skin to increase sweating and heat loss. High temperatures also activate **cholinergic sympathetic fibres** to these areas of the skin. These stimulate sweating, leading to the local formation of **bradykinin**, which further promotes vasodilatation. The flow of blood to the skin can increase up to 30-fold with increases in temperature.

Local skin temperature also directly affects cutaneous blood vessels, which dilate to heat and constrict as temperature falls. Prolonged cold however causes a paradoxical vasodilatation. Cutaneous vessels are also constricted by the baroreceptor reflex, helping to increase TPR and shift blood to the vital organs during haemorrhage or shock.

Cerebral circulation

The brain receives about 15% of cardiac output. The **basilar** and **internal carotid arteries** entering the cranium join to form an arterial ring, the **circle of Willis**, from which arise the **anterior**, **middle** and **posterior cerebral arteries** that supply the cranium (Fig. 24.1b). This arrangement helps to defend the cerebral blood supply, which if occluded causes immediate unconsciousness and irreversible tissue damage within minutes.

The brain, especially the neuronal grey matter, has a very high capillary density (~3000–4000 capillaries/mm³), and *arteriolar autoregulation* is highly developed, allowing cerebral bloodflow to be maintained constant at arterial pressures between about 50 and 170 mmHg. Autoregulation is both myogenic and metabolic; the **K+** and **CO2** concentrations in the surrounding brain are particularly important in causing functional hyperaemia (see Chapter 22). The effect of CO_2 is in part caused by NO release from endothelial cells. Hyperventilation, which reduces arterial CO_2, can cause a marked cerebral vasoconstriction and temporary unconsciousness. Sympathetic regulation of the bloodflow to the brain is probably of minor importance.

The brain and spinal cord float in the **cerebrospinal fluid** (CSF), which is contained within the rigid cranium and the spinal canal. Because the cranium is rigid and its contents are incompressible, the volume of blood within the brain remains roughly constant, and increases in arterial inflow are compensated for by decreases in venous volume. By increasing the tissue mass, brain tumours increase the intracerebral pressure and reduce cerebral bloodflow. Increased intracerebral pressure is partially compensated for by the **Cushing reflex**, a characteristic rise in arterial pressure associated with a reflex bradycardia.

25 The pulmonary and fetal circulations

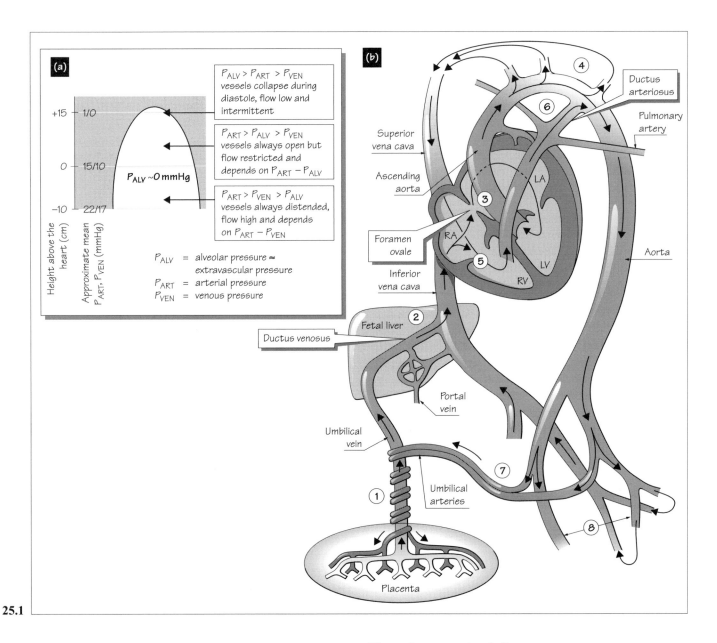

25.1

The lungs contain two circulations. The **bronchial circulation** arises from the aorta, comprises about 1% of cardiac output, and supplies the metabolic needs of the airways. It drains partly into the superior vena cava through bronchial veins, and partly into pulmonary veins. The **pulmonary circulation** receives the entire output of the right ventricle. Its high-density capillary network surrounds the lung alveoli, allowing the O_2-poor blood from the pulmonary arteries to exchange CO_2 for O_2. The pulmonary veins return highly oxygenated blood to the left atrium. The pulmonary circulation contains about 800 ml of blood in recumbent subjects, falling to about 450 ml during quiet standing.

The pulmonary circulation

Mean pulmonary arterial pressure is ~15 mmHg, and left atrial pressure is ~5 mmHg. The right ventricle is able to drive its entire output through the pulmonary circulation utilizing a pressure head of only 10 mmHg, because the resistance of the pulmonary circulation is only 10–15% that of the systemic circulation. This arises because the vessels of the pulmonary microcirculation are short and relatively wide bore, with little resting tone. They are also very numerous, so that their total cross-section is similar to that of the systemic circulation. The walls of both arteries and veins are thin and distensible, and contain comparatively little smooth muscle.

The low pressure within the pulmonary circulation means that regional perfusion of the lungs in the upright position is greatly affected by gravity (Fig. 25.1a). The extravascular pressure throughout the lungs is similar to the alveolar pressure (~0 mmHg). However, the intravascular pressure is low in the lung apices, which are above the heart, and high in the lung bases, which are below the heart. Pulmonary vessels in the lung apices therefore collapse during diastole, causing intermittent flow. Conversely, vessels in the bases of the lungs are perfused throughout the cardiac cycle, and are distended. A small increase in pulmonary arterial pressure during exercise is sufficient to open up apical capillaries, allowing more O_2 uptake by the blood.

The low hydrostatic pressure in pulmonary capillaries (mean of 7–10 mmHg) does not lead to net fluid reabsorption, because it is balanced by a low extravascular hydrostatic pressure (approx −4 mmHg), and an unusually high interstitial plasma protein oncotic pressure (approx 18 mmHg). The lung capillaries therefore produce a small net flow of lymph, which is drained by an extensive pulmonary lymphatic network. During left ventricular failure or mitral stenosis, however, the increased left atrial pressure backs up into the pulmonary circulation, increasing fluid filtration and leading to **pulmonary oedema**.

Neither the sympathetic nervous system nor myogenic/metabolic autoregulation play a role in regulating pulmonary vascular resistance or flow. The pulmonary vasculature is, however, well supplied with sympathetic nerves. When stimulated, these decrease the compliance of the vessels, limiting the pulmonary blood volume so that more blood is available to the systemic circulation.

The most important mechanism regulating pulmonary vascular tone is **hypoxic pulmonary vasoconstriction** (HPV), a process by which pulmonary vessels *constrict* in response to alveolar **hypoxia**. This unique mechanism (*systemic* vessels typically *dilate* to hypoxia) diverts blood away from poorly ventilated regions of the lungs, thereby maximizing the **ventilation–perfusion ratio**. HPV is probably caused by the release of an unidentified endothelial-constricting factor. Hypoxia-mediated inhibition of smooth muscle K^+-channel activity, resulting in membrane depolarization, may also be involved.

The fetal circulation

A diagram of the fetal circulation is shown in Fig. 25.1(b). The fetus receives O_2 and nutrients from, and discharges CO_2 and metabolic waste products into, the maternal circulation. This exchange occurs in the **placenta**, a thick spongy pancake-shaped structure lying between the fetus and the uterine wall. The placenta is composed of a space containing maternal blood, which is packed with **fetal villi**, branching tree-like structures containing fetal arteries, capillaries, and veins. They receive the fetal blood from branches of the two **umbilical arteries**, and drain back into the fetus via the **umbilical vein**. Gas and nutrient exchange occurs between the fetal capillaries in the villi and the maternal blood surrounding and bathing the villi.

The fetal circulation differs from that of adults in that *the right and left ventricles pump the blood in parallel rather than in series*. This arrangement allows the heart and head to receive more highly oxygenated blood, and is made possible by three structural *shunts* unique to the fetus, the **ductus venosus**, the **foramen ovale**, and the **ductus arteriosus** (highlighted in Fig. 25.1b).

Blood leaving the placenta (**1**) via the umbilical vein is 80% saturated with O_2. About half of this flows into the fetus' liver. The rest is diverted into the inferior vena cava via the **ductus venosus** (**2**), mixing with poorly oxygenated venous blood returning from the fetus' lower body. When the resulting relatively oxygen rich mixture (about 67% saturated) enters the right atrium, most of it does not pass into the right ventricle as it would in the adult, but is directed into the left atrium via the **foramen ovale**, an opening between the fetal atria (**3**). Blood then flows into the left ventricle, and is pumped into the ascending aorta, from which it perfuses the head, the coronary circulation, and the arms (**4**). Venous blood from these areas re-enters the heart via the superior vena cava. This blood, now about 35% saturated with O_2, mixes with the fraction of blood from the inferior vena cava not entering the foramen ovale (**5**), and flows into the right ventricle, which pumps it into the pulmonary artery. Instead of then entering the lungs, as it would in the adult, about 90% of the blood leaving the right ventricle is diverted into the descending aorta through the **ductus arteriosus** (**6**). This occurs because pressure in the pulmonary circulation is higher than that in the systemic circulation, as a result of pulmonary vasoconstriction and the collapsed state of the lungs. About 60% of blood entering the descending aorta then flows back to the placenta for oxygenation (**7**). The rest, now 58% saturated with O_2, supplies the fetus' trunk and legs (**8**).

Circulatory changes at birth

Two events at birth quickly cause the fetal circulation to assume a quasi-adult pattern. First, the pulmonary vascular pressure falls well below the systemic pressure because of the initiation of breathing and the resulting pulmonary vasodilatation. Together with constriction of the ductus arteriosus caused by increased blood O_2 levels, this reversal of the pulmonary:systemic pressure gradient, which is aided by the loss of the low-resistance placental circulation, abolishes the bloodflow from the pulmonary artery into the aorta within 30 min after delivery.

Second, tying off the umbilical cord stops venous return from the placenta, abruptly lowering inferior vena caval pressure. Together with the fall in pulmonary resistance, this lowers right atrial pressure, causing within hours functional closure of the foramen ovale. The ductus venosus also closes with the abolition of venous return from the placenta.

Although these fetal circulatory shunts are *functionally* closed soon after birth, complete *structural* closure only occurs after several months. In 20% of adults, the structural closure of the foramen ovale remains incomplete, although this is of no haemodynamic consequence.

26 Cardiovascular reflexes

Intrinsic cardiovascular reflexes

Receptors/reflex/location	Stimulated by	Response activated
Arterial baroreceptors carotid sinus and aortic arch	Change in arterial blood pressure, affects degree of stretch of arterial wall	If pressure decreases: vagal and sympathetic tachycardia; sympathetic vasoconstriction; renin release. If pressure increases: opposite effects

Cardiopulmonary receptors
    atrial mechanoreceptors/Bainbridge reflex
 	
    atrial nonmyelinated vagal efferents
 	
    ventricular and coronary nonmyelinated vagal efferents
	Change in blood volume and pressure in central thoracic compartment; affects degree of stretch of atria, ventricles, coronary arteries	Net effect:
		if volume/pressure decrease: sympathetic and/or vagal tachycardia; vasoconstriction; venoconstriction; reduced production of urine
		if volume/pressure increase: opposite effects

ventricular chemoreceptors/ Bezold–Jarisch effect	Cardiac ischaemia, some drugs	Bradycardia; vasodilatation
J-receptors/lung	Marked lung inflation, pulmonary congestion	Tachycardia; vasodilatation
Arterial chemoreceptors carotid sinus and aortic arch	Severe hypotension, hypoxia, asphyxia causing decreased PO_2, increased PCO_2 and H^+ in blood	Sympathetic vasoconstriction; indirect tachycardia; stimulation of respiration
CNS ischaemic response/Cushing reflex	Brainstem ischaemia	Sympathetic peripheral vasoconstriction

26.1

The cardiovascular system is centrally regulated by **autonomic reflexes**. These work with local mechanisms (see Chapter 22) to minimize fluctuations in the mean arterial blood pressure (MABP) and to maintain adequate perfusion of each organ. **Intrinsic** reflexes respond to stimuli originating from within the cardiovascular system. These include the **baroreceptor**, **cardiopulmonary** and **chemoreceptor** reflexes, and their properties are summarized in Fig. 26.1. Less important **extrinsic** reflexes mediate the cardiovascular response to stimuli originating elsewhere (e.g. pain, temperature changes).

Reflexes involve three components:
1 afferent nerves sense a change in the state of the system, and communicate this to the brain, which
2 processes this information and implements an appropriate response, by
3 altering the activity of efferent nerves controlling cardiac and vascular function, thereby causing homeostatic responses which reverse the change in state.

Intrinsic cardiovascular reflexes
The baroreceptor reflex
This reflex acts rapidly to minimize moment-to-moment fluctuations in the MABP. **Baroreceptors** are afferent (sensory) nerve endings in the walls of the **carotid sinuses** (thin-walled dilatations at the origins of the internal carotid arteries) and the **aortic arch**. These **mechanoreceptors** sense alterations in wall stretch caused by pressure changes, and respond by modifying the frequency at which they fire action potentials. Pressure elevations increase impulse frequency; pressure decreases have the opposite effect.

When MABP decreases, the fall in baroreceptor impulse frequency causes the brain to reduce the firing of vagal efferents supplying the sinoatrial node, thus causing tachycardia. Simultaneously, the activity of sympathetic nerves innervating most blood vessels is increased, causing vasoconstriction. Stimulation of renal sympathetic nerves increases renin release, and consequently angiotensin II production and aldosterone secretion. The resulting tachycardia, vasoconstriction and fluid retention act together to raise MABP. Opposite effects occur when arterial blood pressure rises. The baroreceptors quickly show partial *adaptation* to new pressure levels. Therefore alterations in frequency are greatest while pressure is changing, and tend to moderate when a new steady-state pressure level is established. If unable to prevent MABP from changing to a new level, the reflex will within several hours become *reset* to maintain pressure around this level. It therefore plays little part in long-term regulation of MABP.

There are two types of baroreceptors. *A fibres* have large, myelinated axons, and are activated over lower levels of pressure. *C fibres* have small, unmyelinated axons and respond over higher levels of pressure. Together, these provide an input to the brain, which is most sensitive to pressure changes between

80 and 150 mmHg. Increases in the *pulse pressure* render the baroreceptors more sensitive to changes in MABP.

The brain is able to reset the baroreflex to allow increases in MABP to occur, e.g. during static exercise and the defence reaction. Ageing, hypertension and atherosclerosis decrease arterial wall compliance, reducing baroreceptor reflex sensitivity.

Cardiopulmonary reflexes

Diverse intrinsic cardiovascular reflexes originate in the heart and lungs. Cutting the vagal afferent fibres that mediate these **cardiopulmonary reflexes** causes an increased heart rate and vasoconstriction, especially in skeletal muscle, renal and mesenteric vascular beds. The *net* effect of the cardiopulmonary reflexes is therefore thought to be a **tonic depression** of the *heart rate* and *vascular tone*. The receptors for these reflexes are located mainly (but not entirely) in *low-pressure regions* of the cardiovascular system, and are well placed to sense the *blood volume* in the central thoracic compartment. These reflexes are thought to be particularly important in controlling blood volume and vascular tone, and act together with the baroreceptors to stabilize the blood pressure. However, these reflexes have been studied mainly in animals, and their specific individual roles in humans are incompletely understood.

The best-defined cardiopulmonary reflex is initiated by mechanoreceptors with myelinated vagal afferents, which are located mainly at the juncture of the atria and great veins. These respond to increased atrial volume and pressure by causing a sympathetically mediated tachycardia (the **Bainbridge reflex**). This reflex also helps to control blood volume; its activation decreases the secretion of **antidiuretic hormone** (vasopressin), **cortisol** and **renin**, causing a diuresis.

Other cardiopulmonary reflexes are less well defined:

1 Atrial mechanoreceptors with nonmyelinated vagal afferents respond to increased atrial volume/pressure by causing bradycardia and vasodilatation. The physiological role of this reflex remains obscure.

2 Mechanoreceptors in the left ventricle and coronary arteries with mainly nonmyelinated vagal afferents respond to increased ventricular diastolic pressure and afterload by causing a vasodilatation.

3 Ventricular chemoreceptors are stimulated by substances such as bradykinin and prostaglandins released during cardiac ischaemia. These receptors activate the **coronary chemoreflex**. This response, also called the **Bezold–Jarisch effect**, occurs after the IV injection of many drugs, and involves marked bradycardia and widespread vasodilatation.

Marked lung inflation, especially if oedema is present, activates **juxtapulmonary receptors** ('J' receptors), causing tachycardia and vasodilatation.

Chemoreceptor reflexes

Chemoreceptors activated by **hypoxia**, **hypocapnia**, and **acidosis** are located in the aortic arch and carotid sinuses. These receptors are stimulated during asphyxia, hypoxia, and severe hypotension.

The resulting **chemoreceptor reflex** is mainly involved in stimulating breathing, but also has cardiovascular effects. These include sympathetic constriction of (mainly skeletal muscle) arterioles, splanchnic venoconstriction, and a tachycardia resulting indirectly from the increased lung inflation. This reflex is important because its effects help maintain the bloodflow to the brain at arterial pressures too low to activate the baroreceptors.

The CNS ischaemic response

A powerful generalized peripheral vasoconstriction is stimulated by brainstem hypoxia. This response develops during severe hypotension, helping to maintain the flow of blood to the brain during shock. It also causes the **Cushing reflex**, in which vasoconstriction and hypertension develop when increased cerebrospinal fluid pressure, e.g. due to a brain tumour, produces brainstem hypoxia.

Extrinsic reflexes

Stimuli that are external to the cardiovascular system also exert effects on the heart and vasculature via extrinsic reflexes. Moderate pain causes tachycardia and increases MABP; however, severe pain has the opposite effects. Cold causes cutaneous and coronary vasoconstriction, possibly precipitating angina in susceptible individuals.

Central regulation of cardiovascular reflexes

The view that the brainstem contains a specific **vasomotor centre** responsible for controlling cardiovascular aspects of autonomic function is obsolete. It is now known that cardiovascular autonomic control arises as a result of interactions between areas of the brainstem, the hypothalamus, the cerebral cortex, and the cerebellum.

The afferent nerves carrying impulses from cardiovascular receptors terminate in the **nucleus tractus solitarius** (NTS) of the medulla. Neurons from the NTS project to areas of the brainstem which control both parasympathetic and sympathetic outflow, influencing their level of activation. The **nucleus ambiguus** and **dorsal motor nucleus** contain the cell bodies of the preganglionic vagal parasympathetic neurons, which slow the heart when the cardiovascular receptors report an increased blood pressure to the NTS. Neurons from the NTS also project to areas of **ventrolateral medulla**, from these descend bulbospinal fibres which influence the firing of the sympathetic preganglionic neurons in the IML columns of the spinal cord.

These neural circuits are capable of mediating the basic cardiovascular reflexes. However, the NTS, the other brainstem centres and the IML neurons receive descending inputs from the hypothalamus, which in turn is influenced by impulses from the limbic system of the cerebral cortex. Input from these higher centres modifies the activity of the brainstem centres, allowing the generation of integrated responses in which the functions of the cardiovascular system and other organs are coordinated in such a way that the appropriate responses to changing conditions can be orchestrated.

27 Autonomic control of the cardiovascular system

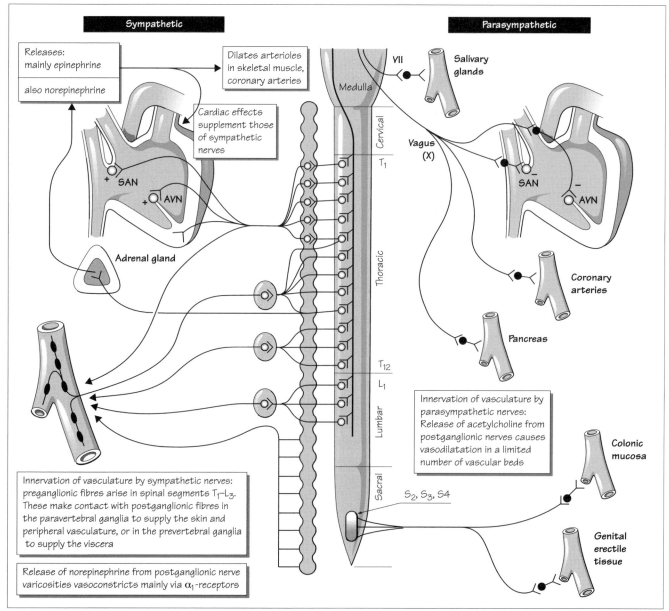

27.1

The **autonomic nervous system** (ANS) comprises a *system of efferent nerves* that regulate the involuntary functioning of most organs, including the heart and vasculature. The cardiovascular effects of the ANS are deployed for two purposes.

First, the ANS provides the effector arm of the cardiovascular *reflexes*, which responds mainly to activation of receptors in the cardiovascular system (see Chapter 26). They are designed to maintain a *constant blood pressure* and adequate tissue perfusion, and they play a crucial role in homeostatic adjustments to *postural changes* (see Chapter 21), *haemorrhage* (see Chapter 30), and *changes in blood gases*.

Second, ANS function is also regulated by signals initiated within the brain as it reacts to *environmental stimuli* or *emotional stress*. The brain can selectively modify or override the cardiovascular reflexes, producing specific patterns of cardiovascular adjustments, which are sometimes coupled with behavioural responses. Complex responses of this type are involved in *exercise* (see Chapter 29), *thermoregulation* (see Chapter 24), the '*fight or flight*' (*defence*) response, and '*playing dead*'.

The ANS is divided into **sympathetic** and **parasympathetic** branches. The nervous pathways of both branches of the ANS consist of two sets of neurons arranged in series. **Preganglionic** neurons originate in the central nervous system and terminate in peripheral **ganglia**, where they synapse with **postganglionic neurons** innervating the target organs.

The sympathetic system

Sympathetic preganglionic neurons originate in the **intermediolateral** (IML) columns of the spinal cord. These neurons exit the spinal cord through ventral roots of segments T_1–L_2, and synapse with the postganglionic fibres in either *paravertebral* or *prevertebral* ganglia. The ganglionic neurotransmitter is **acetylcholine**, and it activates postganglionic **nicotinic cholinergic** receptors. The postganglionic fibres terminate in the effector organs, where they release **norepinephrine**. Preganglionic sympathetic fibres also control the **adrenal medulla**, which releases **epinephrine** and norepinephrine into the blood. Under physiological conditions, the effect of neuronal norepinephrine release is more important than that of epinephrine and norepinephrine released by the adrenal medulla.

Epinephrine and norepinephrine are *catecholamines*, and activate **adrenergic** receptors in the effector organs. These receptors are *G-protein linked* and exist as three types:
- α_1-**receptors** are linked to G_q and have subtypes α_{1A}, α_{1B}, and α_{1D}. Epinephrine and norepinephrine activate α_1-receptors with similar potencies.
- α_2-**receptors** are linked to $G_{i/o}$ and have subtypes α_{2A}, α_{2B}, and α_{2C}. Epinephrine activates α_2-receptors more potently than does norepinephrine.
- β-**receptors** are linked to G_s and have subtypes β_1, β_2, and β_3. Norepinephrine is more potent than epinephrine at β_1- and β_3-receptors, while epinephrine is more potent at β_2-receptors.

Effects on the heart

Catecholamines acting via cardiac β_1-**receptors** have positive inotropic and chronotropic effects via mechanisms described in Chapter 11. At rest, cardiac sympathetic nerves exert a tonic accelerating influence on the sinoatrial node, which is however overshadowed by the opposite and dominant effect of parasympathetic vagal tone.

Effects on the vasculature

At rest, vascular sympathetic nerves fire impulses at a rate of 1–2 impulses/s, thereby tonically vasoconstricting the arteries, arterioles, and veins. Increasing activation of the sympathetic system causes further vasoconstriction. Vasoconstriction is mediated mainly by α_1-**receptors** on the vascular smooth muscle cells. The arterial system, particularly the arterioles, is more densely innervated by the sympathetic system than is the venous system. Sympathetic vasoconstriction is particularly marked in the splanchnic, renal, cutaneous and skeletal muscle vascular beds.

The vasculature also contains both β_1- and β_2-receptors, which when stimulated exert a *vasodilating* influence, especially in the *skeletal* and *coronary* circulations. These may play a limited role in dilating these vascular beds in response to epinephrine release, for example during mental stress. In some species, sympathetic *cholinergic* fibres innervate skeletal muscle blood vessels and cause vasodilatation during the defence reaction. A similar but minor role for such nerves in man has been proposed, but is unproven.

It is a common fallacy that the sympathetic nerves are always activated *en masse*. In reality, changes in sympathetic vasoconstrictor activity can be limited to certain regions (e.g. to the skin during thermoregulation). Similarly, a sympathetically mediated tachycardia occurs with no change in inotropy or vascular resistance during the Bainbridge reflex (see Chapter 26).

The parasympathetic system

The parasympathetic preganglionic neurons involved in regulating the heart have their cell bodies in the **nucleus ambiguus** and the **dorsal motor nucleus** of the medulla. Their axons run in the **vagus** nerve (cranial nerve X), and release acetylcholine onto nicotinic receptors on short postganglionic neurons originating in the cardiac plexus. These innervate the *sinoatrial (SAN)* and *atrioventricular nodes (AVN)*, and the *atria*.

Effects on the heart

Basal acetylcholine release by vagal nerve terminals acts on muscarinic receptors to slow cardiac pacemaking tonically by the SAN. Increased vagal tone further decreases the heart rate and the speed of impulse conduction through the AVN and also decreases the force of atrial contraction when activated (see also Chapter 10).

Effects on the vasculature

Although vagal slowing of the heart can decrease the blood pressure by lowering cardiac output, the parasympathetic system has no effect on total peripheral resistance, because it innervates only a limited number of vascular beds. Activation of parasympathetic fibres in the pelvic nerve causes **erection** by vasodilating arterioles in the erectile tissue of the genitalia. Parasympathetic nerves also cause vasodilatation in the pancreas and salivary glands.

28 The control of blood volume

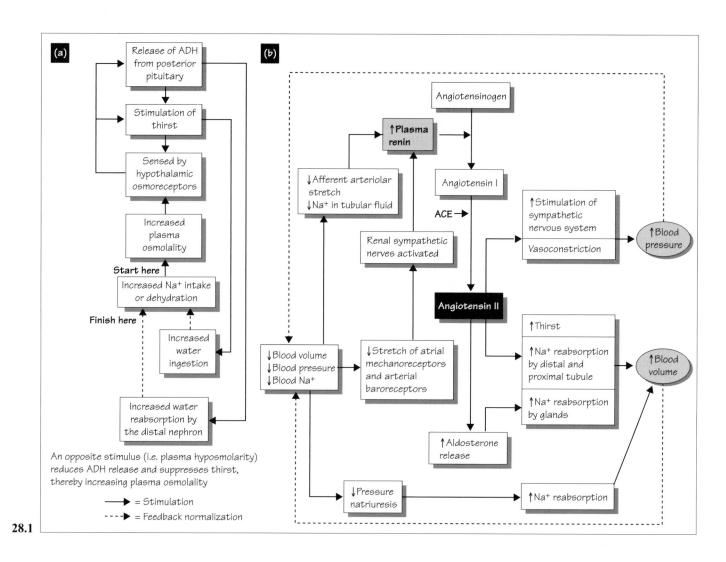

28.1

The baroreceptor system effectively minimizes short-term fluctuations in the arterial blood pressure. Over the longer term, however, the ability of the body to sustain a constant blood pressure depends on the maintenance of a *constant blood volume*. This dependency arises because alterations in the blood volume affect venous return and therefore cardiac output, one of the major determinants of arterial blood pressure.

The volume of the blood is affected by changes in the total body contents of both Na+ and water. Both of these parameters are mainly controlled by the kidneys. The maintenance of a stable blood pressure therefore involves mechanisms that adjust renal excretion of sodium and water, so that the contents of both remain unchanged.

Plasma volume: the role of sodium and osmoregulation

Alterations in the water content of the body, caused for example by variations in fluid intake or perspiration, result in changes in

the plasma **osmolality**. The osmolality of a solution is defined as the total concentration of osmotically active particles per kilogram of water.

Any deviation of plasma osmolality from its normal value of *~290 mOsmol/kg* is sensed by *hypothalamic osmoreceptors*, which activate the homeostatic feedback control system illustrated in Fig. 28.1(a). The osmoreceptors regulate both thirst and the release from the posterior pituitary gland of **antidiuretic hormone (ADH**, also **vasopressin)**, a peptide which suppresses renal water excretion. For example, dehydration raises plasma osmolality. This results in an increased thirst, and also enhances the release of ADH. ADH acts on the distal nephron to increase its reabsorption of water, thereby reducing the loss of water in the urine. Both effects act to bring plasma osmolality back to its set point by restoring the water content of the body. The opposite effects are stimulated by an excess of body water, which reduces plasma osmolality.

An important consequence of this osmoregulatory mechanism is that the plasma volume is primarily controlled by the Na+ content of the extracellular fluid (ECF). Na+ and its associated anions Cl- and HCO_3^- account for about 95% of the osmotic solute present in the ECF, of which the plasma is a part. Any change in the Na+ content of the body (e.g. after eating a salty meal) will quickly affect plasma osmolality. This will cause the osmoregulatory system to readjust the body water content (and therefore the plasma volume) in order to restore the plasma osmolality. Under normal conditions, therefore, alterations in body Na+ lead to changes in plasma volume. It follows that the maintenance of a stable plasma volume requires the tight regulation of the ECF Na+ content, a function mainly carried out by the kidneys.

Control of plasma volume by the kidneys

As shown in Fig. 28.1(b), changes in vascular volume and pressure activate several mechanisms. These mechanisms cause compensatory alterations in renal Na+ excretion which return these parameters back to their original levels. Only effects of decreases in vascular volume and pressure are illustrated; however, increases in these parameters cause opposite compensatory responses.

Pressure natriuresis is an intrinsic renal homeostatic mechanism by which decreases in blood volume and pressure strongly inhibit diuresis and natriuresis (Na+ excretion in the urine). Although the mechanisms of pressure natriuresis remain imperfectly understood, it is thought that decreases in renal perfusion pressure cause a fall in the hydrostatic pressure within the renal interstitium surrounding the proximal tubule. This promotes the reabsorption of fluid from the nephron, acting to restore the blood volume. Opposite effects occur during volume expansion.

The **renin–angiotensin–aldosterone system** responds to stimuli associated with reductions in vascular volume and pressure by inhibiting Na+ excretion, increasing thirst, and causing vasoconstriction. **Renin** is a proteolytic enzyme stored in the *granular cells* of the renal juxtaglomerular apparatus. Renin release into the blood is increased by:

1 Activation of the baroreceptor reflex by a reduction of vascular pressure, which increases firing of sympathetic nerves innervating the granular cells.
2 Decreased atrial stretch/pressure, sensed by cardiac mechanoreceptors.
3 Decreased stretch of renal afferent arterioles caused by a fall in renal perfusion pressure.
4 The release of prostacyclin (PGI_2) by the *macula densa cells* of the early distal tubule. The macula densa cells, which form part of the juxtaglomerular apparatus, are stimulated to release PGI_2 by a fall in the NaCl content of the tubular fluid.

Once released, renin cleaves a plasma α_2-globulin, **angiotensinogen**, liberating the decapeptide **angiotensin I**. Plasma angiotensin I is then acted on by **angiotensin-converting enzyme** (ACE) on the surface of endothelial cells, giving rise to the **octapeptide angiotensin II**. Angiotensin II has a variety of effects, which raise blood pressure and volume. These include increasing Na+ reabsorption by the proximal tubule, stimulating thirst, promoting ADH release, increasing the activation of the sympathetic nervous system, and causing a direct vasoconstriction. ACE, also called **kininase II**, has the additional function of breaking down bradykinin, a vasodilating local hormone.

Angiotensin II also promotes the release of the steroid hormone **aldosterone** from the zona glomerulosa cells of the adrenal cortex. Aldosterone increases Na+ retention by acting on the principal cells of the distal nephron to enhance Na+ reabsorption. It does so by increasing the synthesis of both Na+ pumps in the basolateral membrane and Na+ channels in the apical membrane of these cells. In addition, aldosterone conserves body Na+ by enhancing its reabsorption from several types of glands, including the salivary and sweat glands. Aldosterone secretion is also increased by decreased stimulation of the atrial volume/pressure mechanoreceptors.

Atrial natriuretic peptide (ANP) is a 28-amino-acid peptide released from atrial myocytes when they are stretched by an increased atrial volume. ANP can cause both diuresis and natriuresis by increasing the glomerular filtration rate, decreasing renin and aldosterone secretion, and reducing Na+ reabsorption throughout the nephron. ANP also dilates arterioles and increases capillary permeability. On a cellular level, ANP stimulates a membrane-associated guanylyl cyclase, raising the intracellular cyclic GMP concentration. ANP may be involved in the homeostatic response to volume overload, although its precise physiological role is controversial.

Antidiuretic hormone in volume regulation

Under emergency conditions, plasma volume is maintained at the expense of osmoregulation. For example, a fall in vascular volume sensed by atrial pressure/stretch mechanoreceptors causes an increased ADH release, leading to water retention by the kidneys. In addition, the ADH system is rendered more sensitive to increases in plasma osmolality by a fall in vascular volume, so that ADH release is promoted even at normal plasma osmolality (Fig. 28.1a). Increases in plasma volume have the opposite effect on ADH release.

29 Cardiovascular effects of exercise

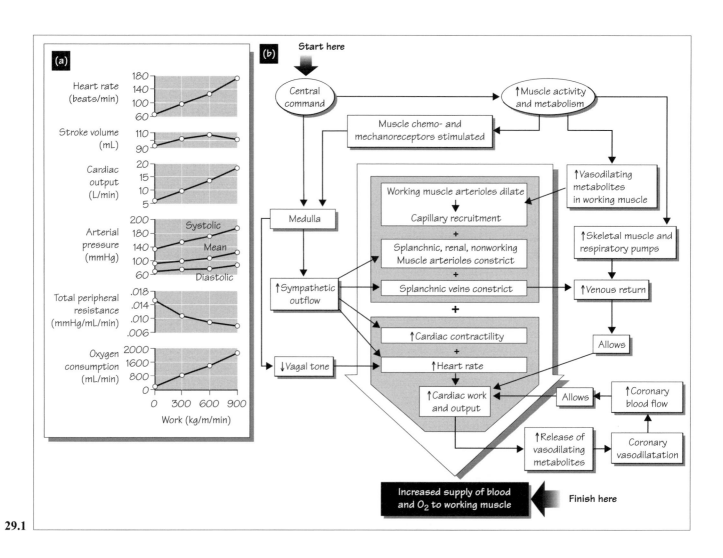

29.1

Figure 29.1(a) summarizes important cardiovascular adaptations which occur at increasing levels of dynamic (rhythmic) exercise, thereby allowing working muscles to be supplied with the increased amount of O_2 they require. By far the most important of these is an increase in cardiac output (CO), which rises almost linearly with the rate of muscle O_2 consumption (level of work) as a result of increases in both *heart rate* and to a lesser extent *stroke volume*. The heart rate is accelerated by a reduction in vagal tone, and by increases in sympathetic nerve firing and circulating catecholamines. The resulting stimulation of cardiac β-adrenoceptors increases stroke volume by *increasing myocardial contractility* and enabling more complete systolic emptying of the ventricles.

Table 29.1 shows that the increased CO is channelled mainly to the active muscles, which may receive 85% of CO, against about 15–20% at rest, and to the heart. This is caused by a profound arteriolar vasodilatation in these organs. Dilatation of precapillary sphincters causes **capillary recruitment**, a large increase in the number of open capillaries, which shortens the diffusion distance between capillaries and muscle fibres. This, combined with increases in P_{CO_2}, temperature and acidity, promotes the release of O_2 from haemoglobin, allowing skeletal muscle to increase its O_2 extraction from the basal level of 25–30% to about 90% during maximal exercise.

Increased firing of sympathetic nerves and levels of circulating catecholamines constrict arterioles in the *splanchnic* and *renal* vascular beds, and in *nonexercising muscle*, reducing the bloodflow to these organs. Cutaneous bloodflow is also initially reduced. As core body temperature rises, however, cutaneous bloodflow increases as autonomically mediated vasodilatation occurs to promote cooling (see Chapter 24). With very strenuous exercise, cutaneous perfusion again falls as vasoconstriction diverts blood to the muscles. The increased CO causes a rise in venous return. Venous return is enhanced by increased activity

Table 29.1 Cardiac output and regional blood flow in a sedentary man. Values are ml/min.

	Quiet standing	Exercise
Cardiac output	5900	24000
Blood flow to:		
Heart	250	1000
Brain	750	750
Active skeletal muscle	650	20850
Inactive skeletal muscle	650	300
Skin	500	500
Kidney, liver, gastrointestinal tract, etc.	3100	600

of skeletal muscle and respiratory pumps, and is also transiently promoted by splanchnic constriction, which reduces the capacitance of the venous system. Bloodflow to the crucial cerebral vasculature remains constant.

Vasodilatation of the skeletal and cutaneous vascular beds decreases in total peripheral resistance. This is sufficient to balance the effect of the increased CO on diastolic blood pressure, which rises only slightly and may even fall, depending on the balance between skeletal muscle vasodilatation and splanchnic/renal vasoconstriction. Significant rises in the systolic and pulse pressures are, however, caused by the more rapid and forceful ejection of blood by the left ventricle, leading to some elevation of the mean arterial blood pressure.

Effects of exercise on plasma volume

Arteriolar dilatation in skeletal muscles increases capillary hydrostatic pressure, while capillary recruitment vastly increases the surface area of the microcirculation available to exchange fluid. These effects, coupled with a rise in interstitial osmolarity caused by an increased production of metabolites within the muscle fibres, lead via the Starling mechanism to *extravasation of fluid into muscles*. Taking into account also fluid losses caused by sweating, plasma volume may decrease by 15% during strenuous exercise. This fluid loss is partially compensated by enhanced fluid reabsorption in the vasoconstricted vascular beds, where capillary pressure decreases.

Regulation and coordination of the cardiovascular adaptation to exercise

In anticipation of exercise, and during its initial stages, a process termed **central command** (Fig. 29.1b, upper left) causes the cardiovascular adaptations necessary for increased effort. Impulses from the cerebral cortex act on the medulla to suppress vagal tone, thereby increasing the heart rate and CO. Central command is also thought to decrease the sensitivity of the baroreceptor reflex to blood pressure. This results in an increased sympathetic outflow which contributes to the rise in CO and causes constriction of the splanchnic and renal circulations. An increase in circulating epinephrine also vasodilates

skeletal muscle arterioles via β_2-receptors. The magnitude of these anticipatory effects increases in proportion to the degree of perceived effort.

Central command is thought to dominate cardiovascular regulation during mild exercise. In moderate or strenuous exercise, however, two further control systems are activated which become crucial. These involve: (i) autonomic reflexes (Fig. 29.1b, left); and (ii) direct effects of metabolites generated locally in working skeletal and cardiac muscle (right).

Systemic effects mediated by autonomic reflexes

Nervous impulses originating mainly from receptors in working muscle which respond to contraction (mechanoreceptors) and locally generated metabolites and ischaemia (chemoreceptors) are carried to the CNS via afferent nerves. CNS autonomic control centres respond by suppressing vagal tone and causing graded increases in sympathetic outflow which are matched to the ongoing level of exercise. An increased release of epinephrine and norepinephrine from the adrenal glands causes plasma catecholamines to rise by as much as 10–20-fold. These autonomic effects are also promoted by receptors activated by increased respiration.

Effects of local metabolites on muscle and heart

The autonomic reflexes described above are responsible for most of the cardiac and vasoconstricting adaptations to exercise. However, the marked vasodilatation of coronary and skeletal muscle arterioles is almost entirely caused by *local metabolites* generated in the heart and working skeletal muscle. This **metabolic hyperaemia** (Chapter 22) causes decreased vascular resistance and increased bloodflow. Capillary recruitment (see above) is an important consequence of metabolic hyperaemia.

Static exercises such as lifting and carrying involve maintained muscle contractions with no joint movement. This results in vascular compression and a decreased muscle bloodflow, leading to a build up of muscle metabolites. These activate muscle chemoreceptors, resulting in a **pressor reflex** involving *tachycardia*, and *increases CO* and *TPR*. The resulting rise in blood pressure is much greater than in dynamic exercise causing the same rise in O_2 consumption.

Effects of training

Athletic training has effects on the cardiovascular system which improve delivery of O_2 to muscle cells, allowing them to work harder. The ventricular cavities become larger, increasing the stroke volume from about 75 to 120 ml. The resting heart rate may fall as low as 45 beats/min, due to an increase in vagal tone, while the maximal rate remains near 180 beats/min. These changes allow CO to increase more during strenuous exercise, reaching levels of 35 L/min or more. TPR falls, in part due to a decreased sympathetic outflow. The capillary density of skeletal muscle increases, and the muscle fibres contain more mitochondria, promoting oxygen extraction and utilization.

30 Shock and haemorrhage

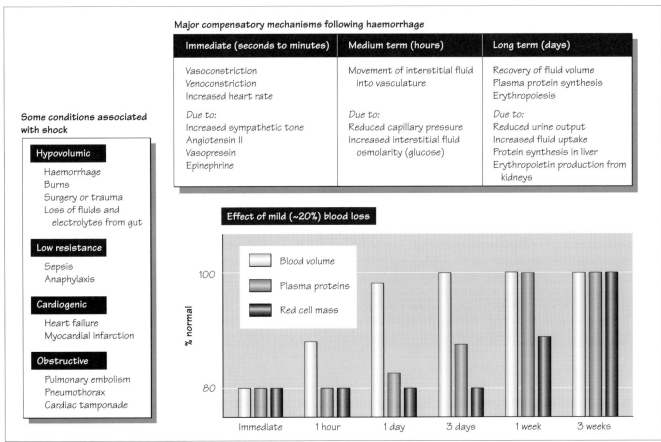

Major compensatory mechanisms following haemorrhage

Immediate (seconds to minutes)	Medium term (hours)	Long term (days)
Vasoconstriction Venoconstriction Increased heart rate	Movement of interstitial fluid into vasculature	Recovery of fluid volume Plasma protein synthesis Erythropoiesis
Due to: Increased sympathetic tone Angiotensin II Vasopressin Epinephrine	Due to: Reduced capillary pressure Increased interstitial fluid osmolarity (glucose)	Due to: Reduced urine output Increased fluid uptake Protein synthesis in liver Erythropoietin production from kidneys

Some conditions associated with shock

Hypovolumic

Haemorrhage
Burns
Surgery or trauma
Loss of fluids and electrolytes from gut

Low resistance

Sepsis
Anaphylaxis

Cardiogenic

Heart failure
Myocardial infarction

Obstructive

Pulmonary embolism
Pneumothorax
Cardiac tamponade

Effect of mild (~20%) blood loss

Blood volume
Plasma proteins
Red cell mass

% normal — 100, 80

Immediate, 1 hour, 1 day, 3 days, 1 week, 3 weeks

30.1

Although the term **shock** is used by the layman to describe a psychological state, clinically it refers to an acute condition where cardiac output is insufficient for adequate perfusion of the tissues. The patient appears pale, grey or cyanotic, with cold clammy skin, a weak, rapid pulse, and rapid shallow breathing. Urine output is reduced, and the blood pressure is generally low, although this may be only relative to the patient's normal blood pressure. Conscious patients may suffer from intense thirst.

Cardiovascular shock may be caused by a reduced blood volume (**hypovolumic shock**), profound vasodilatation (**low-resistance shock**), failure of the heart to maintain output due to cardiac disease (**cardiogenic shock**), or blockage of the cardiopulmonary circuit (**obstructive shock**).

Haemorrhagic shock

Blood loss (**haemorrhage**) is a common cause of hypovolumic shock, and will be used to demonstrate compensatory mechanisms. Loss of up to ~10% of total blood volume does not elicit shock, as adequate perfusion can be maintained. If 20–30% of blood volume is lost, shock is normally induced and blood pressure may be depressed, although death is not common. Loss

of 30–40% of volume, however, causes a profound reduction in blood pressure, with severe shock which may lead to **refractory** or irreversible shock, or other serious complications. Above 50% death is generally inevitable.

Immediate compensation

The baroreceptors detect the fall in blood pressure, sympathetic drive is increased, and parasympathetic drive is decreased. Heart rate rises, and vasoconstriction increases the resistance of the splanchnic, cutaneous, renal and skeletal muscle circulations, increasing total peripheral resistance and supporting blood pressure. Perfusion in these tissues is reduced, leading to pallor, reduced urine production, and lactic acidosis. The increased sympathetic discharge also results in sweating, and the characteristic clammy skin. Sympathetic activity in the kidneys, coupled with reduced renal artery pressure, stimulates the **renin–angiotensin system**, which results in the production of **angiotensin II**, a powerful vasoconstrictor. This plays an important additional role in the initial recovery of blood pressure, and stimulates the feeling of intense thirst. In more severe blood loss the reduction in cardiac stretch receptor output stimulates the production of **vasopressin** (antidiuretic hormone), and epinephrine production by the adrenal glands is increased, both of which contribute to the vasoconstriction. In combination these initial mechanisms may prevent any significant fall in blood pressure following moderate blood loss, even though the degree of shock may be serious.

Medium-term mechanisms

The sympathetic-mediated vasoconstriction leads to a decrease in capillary hydrostatic pressure. The oncotic pressure exerted by plasma proteins is however maintained, resulting in movement of fluid from the interstitial space back into the vasculature (see Chapter 20). This 'internal transfusion' may increase blood volume by ~0.5 L. Increased glucose production by the liver may contribute to this process by raising the osmolarity of plasma and interstitial fluid, and drawing water from the intracellular compartment. However this process results in haemodilution, and so reduces O_2 delivery. Patients with severe shock often present with a reduced haematocrit.

Long-term recovery

Fluid volume is brought back to normal over a day or two by increased fluid intake and decreased fluid loss in the urine. Urine production is decreased by the sympathetic renal vasoconstriction, and stimulation of aldosterone production by angiotensin II causes increased reabsorption of Na^+ in the kidneys, elevating the blood volume. Water reabsorption is also increased by vasopressin. The liver replaces plasma proteins within a week, and the haematocrit returns to normal within a few weeks as a result of stimulation of **erythropoiesis** (see Chapter 6).

Refractory shock (*decompensated or irreversible*) is used to describe the condition of those patients where, after a period of time, cardiac output remains depressed or may decline, even in the face of a replenished blood volume and vasoconstrictor drugs. Refractory shock commonly occurs when blood loss exceeds ~30% and several hours have passed before blood volume is replenished. It can be associated with all types of cardiovascular shock.

Although initially blood pressure may be maintained by the compensatory mechanisms above, after a period of a few hours it may begin to fall, eventually leading to tissue ischaemia. This is of particular importance in the cardiac, cerebral and renal circulations. The fall in blood pressure in the refractory phase is related to a reduction in sympathetic vasoconstriction, leading to vasodilatation, and slowing of heart rate. Previous tissue ischaemia may also have caused damage to the microvasculature, with a consequent increase in permeability. Blood pressure may thus be further compromised by loss of fluid to the tissues.

Late complications of prolonged shock include **renal damage** and the **adult respiratory distress syndrome** (ARDS). ARDS has a very high mortality, and is characterized by acute respiratory failure. It can also be caused by sepsis and trauma.

Other types of hypovolumic shock

Severe burns result in a loss of plasma in the exudate from damaged tissue. Although total blood volume is decreased, because red cells are not lost, there is significant **haemoconcentration**, which will increase blood viscosity. This makes it more difficult for the heart to pump blood through the circulation. The treatment of burns-related shock therefore involves infusion of plasma rather than whole blood.

Traumatic and surgical shock can occur after major injury or surgery. Although partly due to external blood loss, blood and plasma can also be lost into the tissues, and there may be dehydration. Severe tissue damage can also release K^+, free radicals and myoglobin, which may have additional vascular effects and cause further tissue damage. Traumatic shock may result in kidney damage as a result of products from damaged tissues clogging the tubules.

Other conditions and several diseases may result in hypovolumic shock. Severe diarrhoea or vomiting cause loss of Na^+, with a consequent reduction in blood volume even if water is given. An example is **cholera**, where unless replacement electrolytes can be given the blood volume may fall sufficiently for death to occur as a result of shock.

Low-resistance shock

Several types of low-resistance shock also increase vascular permeability, with loss of proteins and fluid to the tissues (see Chapter 20). The condition may therefore be complicated by an added hypovolaemia. Unlike hypovolumic shock, low-resistance shock may present with warm skin as a result of the profound peripheral vasodilatation. In severe cases treatment may require the application of vasoconstrictors, although this may be ineffective if fluid loss to the tissues is too great.

Septic shock

In sepsis, infecting bacteria release **endotoxins**, which cause profound vasodilatation, partly via the induction of **inducible nitric oxide synthase** in various tissues (see Chapter 23). Capillary permeability and cardiac function may also be impaired, with a consequent loss of fluid to the tissues and depressed cardiac output, both of which will contribute to the problem.

Anaphylactic shock

Anaphylactic shock is a rapidly developing and life-threatening condition that can result from the presentation of antigen to a previously sensitized individual, for example a single bee sting. A severe allergic reaction may result, with the release of large amounts of histamine. This in turn causes profound vasodilatation, and an increase in the permeability of the microvasculature, leading to protein and fluid loss, and consequent gross oedema. Rapid application of antihistamines and glucocorticoids is generally required, but in severe reactions the immediate application of epinephrine may save the patient's life, primarily by causing generalized vasoconstriction.

31 Risk factors for cardiovascular disease

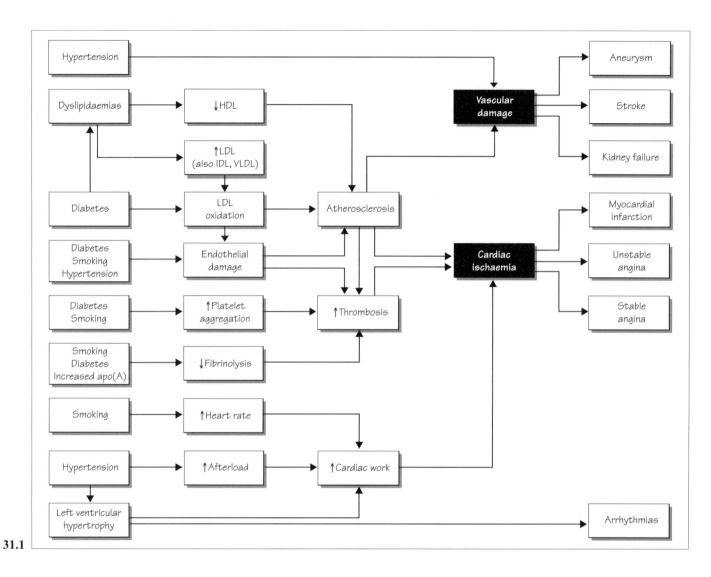

31.1

Cardiovascular *risk factors* are conditions or activities that increase the probability that morbidity (illness) and/or mortality due to cardiovascular disease (CVD) will occur. Risk factors usually act as causes or promotors of CVD. In some cases they are also indicators that subclinical (i.e. as yet symptomless) CVD is already present. Table 31.1 presents an abbreviated summary of the impact of major risk factors on coronary heart disease as determined by the Framingham Heart Study.

Risk factors can be **fixed** or **modifiable**. Fixed risk factors include *age, male sex,* and *family history of CVD*. Modifiable risk factors, including *smoking, dyslipidaemias, hypertension, diabetes mellitus, obesity,* and *physical inactivity*, can be eliminated or ameliorated by lifestyle alteration and/or pharmacological therapy. This approach has been shown to reduce the occurrence and severity of CVD, and is particularly justified because overt CVD is typically both irreversible and ultimately

lethal. Patients often have multiple modifiable risk factors, in which case all of these should be simultaneously targeted.

Figure 31.1 illustrates important mechanisms by which major risk factors promote **vascular damage** and **cardiac ischaemia** (oxygen and nutrient starvation), the two conditions underlying the vast majority of CVD. These mechanisms are described in greater detail in Chapters 33, 34, 36–40, 43 and 45.

Modifiable risk factors

Dyslipidaemias are a heterogeneous group of conditions characterized by abnormal levels of one or more **lipoproteins**. Lipoproteins are blood-borne particles that contain cholesterol and other lipids. They function to transfer lipids between the intestines, liver, and other organs (see Chapter 33).

Dyslipidaemias involving excessive plasma concentrations of **low density lipoprotein**, or **LDL**, are associated with rises in

Table 31.1 Major modifiable risk factors: effects on the risk of coronary heart disease in men and women aged 35–64 years.

Risk factors	Age-adjusted relative risk*	
	Men	Women
Cholesterol > 240 mg/dl	1.9	1.8
Hypertension > 140/90 mmHg	2.0	2.2
Diabetes	1.5	3.7
Left ventricular hypertrophy	3.0	4.6
Smoking	1.5	1.1

* Indicates relative risk for individuals with a given factor vs. those without it.

plasma cholesterol levels, because LDL contains 70% of total plasma cholesterol. As the level of plasma cholesterol rises, particularly above 240 mg/dl (6.2 mmol/L), there is a progressive increase in the risk of CVD due to the attendant rise in LDL levels. LDL plays a pivotal role in causing atherosclerosis because it can be converted to an oxidized form, which damages the vascular wall (Chapter 34). Drugs that lower plasma LDL (and therefore oxidized LDL) slow the progression of atherosclerosis and reduce the occurrence of CVD. Elevated levels of **lipoprotein (a)**, a form of LDL containing the unique protein *apo(a)*, have been reported to confer additional cardiovascular risk. Apo(a) contains a structural component closely resembling plasminogen, and it may inhibit fibrinolysis (see Chapter 7) by competing with plasminogen for endogenous activators.

Conversely, the risk of CVD is *inversely* related to the plasma concentration of **high density lipoprotein (HDL)**, possibly because HDL functions to remove cholesterol from body tissues. The ratio of total : HDL cholesterol is therefore a better predictor of risk than cholesterol levels per se. Low HDL levels often coexist with high levels of plasma *triglycerides*, which are also correlated with CVD. This is probably due to the atherogenicity of the triglyceride-rich **very low density lipoprotein (VLDL)** and **intermediate density lipoprotein (IDL)**.

Diabetes mellitus is a metabolic disease present in approximately 5% of the population. Diabetics either lack the hormone *insulin* entirely, or become resistant to its actions. The latter condition, which usually develops in adulthood, is termed noninsulin-dependent diabetes (NIDDM), and accounts for 95% of diabetics. Diabetes causes progressive damage to both the microvasculature and larger arteries over many years. Approximately 75% of diabetics eventually die from CVD.

There is evidence that NIDDM patients have both endothelial damage and increased levels of oxidized LDL. Both effects may be a result of mechanisms associated with the hyperglycaemia characteristic of this condition. Also, blood coagulability is increased in NIDDM, because of elevated plasminogen activator inhibitor 1 (PAI-1) and increased platelet aggregability. NIDDM is often associated with an atherogenic dyslipidaemia involving high plasma triglycerides (VLDL and IDL) and low HDL. Many dyslipidaemic NIDDM patients are also hypertensive. This clustering of CVD risk factors, all of which may be related to a common metabolic abnormality, is sometimes termed **syndrome X**.

Tobacco smoking causes cardiovascular disease by lowering HDL, increasing blood coagulability, and damaging the endothelium, thereby promoting atherosclerosis. In addition, nicotine-induced cardiac stimulation and a carbon monoxide-mediated reduction of the oxygen-carrying capacity of the blood also occur. These effects, coupled with an increased occurrence of coronary spasm, set the stage for cardiac ischaemia and myocardial infarction. Epidemiological evidence suggests that CVD risk is not reduced with low tar cigarettes.

Hypertension defined as a blood pressure above 140/90 mmHg, occurs in ~25% of the population. Hypertension promotes atherogenesis, probably by damaging the endothelium and causing other deleterious effects on the walls of large arteries. Hypertension damages blood vessels of the brain and kidneys, increasing the risk of stroke and renal failure. The higher cardiac workload imposed by the increased arterial pressure also causes a thickening of the left ventricular wall. This **left ventricular hypertrophy (LVH)** is both a cause and harbinger of more serious cardiovascular damage. LVH predisposes the myocardium to arrhythmias and ischaemia, and is a major contributor to heart failure, myocardial infarction, and sudden death.

Physical inactivity promotes CVD via multiple mechanisms. A low level of fitness is associated with reduced plasma HDL, higher levels of blood pressure and insulin resistance, and **obesity**, itself a CVD risk factor. Studies show that a moderate to high level of fitness is associated with a halving of CVD mortality.

Fixed risk factors
Family history of CVD
Numerous epidemiological surveys have firmly established the existence of a familial predisposition to CVD. This arises in part because many CVD risk factors (e.g. hypertension, diabetes, dyslipidaemias) have a *multifactorial genetic basis* (are due to multiple abnormal genes interacting with environmental influences). Additional deleterious genetic influences are also probably involved, because the familial predisposition remains if epidemiological data are corrected for known risk factors. For example, the angiotensin-converting enzyme (ACE) gene can exist in two forms, characterized by the insertion/deletion of a 287-basepair DNA segment within intron 16. Those homozygous for the deletion polymorphism have higher plasma ACE concentrations, which may modestly increase the risk of suffering myocardial infarction.

Male sex
Middle-aged women are much less likely than men to develop CVD. This difference progressively narrows after the menopause, and is mainly oestrogen mediated. Oestrogen's potentially beneficial actions include acting as an antioxidant, lowering LDL and raising HDL, stimulating the expression and activity of nitric oxide synthase, causing vasodilatation, and increasing the production of plasminogen.

32 Clinical measurement of cardiac and vascular function

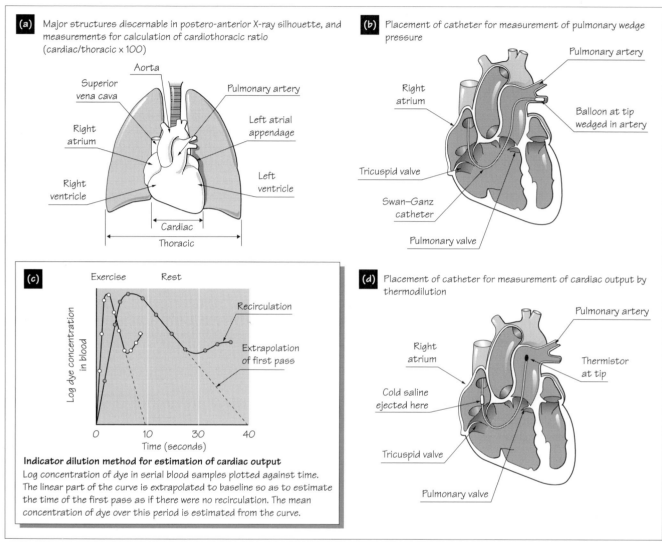

(a) Major structures discernable in postero-anterior X-ray silhouette, and measurements for calculation of cardiothoracic ratio (cardiac/thoracic x 100)

- Aorta
- Superior vena cava
- Pulmonary artery
- Right atrium
- Left atrial appendage
- Right ventricle
- Left ventricle
- Cardiac
- Thoracic

(b) Placement of catheter for measurement of pulmonary wedge pressure

- Pulmonary artery
- Right atrium
- Balloon at tip wedged in artery
- Tricuspid valve
- Swan–Ganz catheter
- Pulmonary valve

(c)

- Exercise
- Rest
- Recirculation
- Extrapolation of first pass
- Log dye concentration in blood
- Time (seconds): 0, 10, 30, 40

Indicator dilution method for estimation of cardiac output
Log concentration of dye in serial blood samples plotted against time. The linear part of the curve is extrapolated to baseline so as to estimate the time of the first pass as if there were no recirculation. The mean concentration of dye over this period is estimated from the curve.

(d) Placement of catheter for measurement of cardiac output by thermodilution

- Pulmonary artery
- Right atrium
- Thermistor at tip
- Cold saline ejected here
- Tricuspid valve
- Pulmonary valve

32.1

General investigations

The arterial pulse, electrocardiogram (ECG) and heart sounds are dealt with in Chapters 13 and 16.

Blood pressure

Measurements are made using a **sphygmomanometer**. This consists of an inflatable cuff around the upper arm over the brachial artery, connected to a pressure gauge. The cuff is inflated until its pressure is greater than systolic pressure, at which point the arteries are compressed and the radial pulse disappears. A stethoscope is placed over the artery just below the cuff, and the cuff pressure slowly reduced. When the pressure falls to the level of the systolic blood pressure, clear sounds are heard (**Korotkoff sounds**). These are due to turbulence as blood is forced through the partially occluded artery. As the cuff pressure declines, the Korotkoff sounds become suddenly muffled, then disappear completely. This cuff pressure is generally taken as diastolic pressure, as it is easiest to recognize. Sometimes the sounds disappear then reappear between the systolic and diastolic pressures, and care should be taken not to confuse these changes with their final disappearance.

Jugular venous pressure

Pressure in the internal jugular vein provides an estimate of right atrial pressure (see Chapter 13). Jugular venous pressure (JVP) is measured in patients positioned at an angle of 30–60°, and is taken as the vertical height between the manubrio-sternal angle and the point at which the vein collapses, i.e. the height of the venous column at end-expiration. JVP is normally less than 3 cm, but is increased when central venous pressure

(CVP) is raised, e.g. **right heart failure**. *Tricuspid regurgitation* (backflow during systole) causes a very large pulse.

X-rays (chest radiography)

An essential diagnostic tool. The initial X-ray is taken in the postero-anterior direction. Figure 32.1(a) shows diagrammatically the major structures in which gross abnormalities can be detected. Heart size and **cardiothoracic ratio** (size of heart relative to thoracic cavity) can also be estimated. This ratio is normally < 50%, except in neonates, infants, and athletes.

Echocardiography and Doppler ultrasound

Echocardiography can be used to detect enlarged hearts and abnormal cardiac movement, and estimate ejection fraction. An ultrasound pulse of ~2.5 MHz is generated by a piezoelectric transmitter-receiver on the chest wall, and reflected back by internal structures. As sound travels through fluid at a known velocity, the time taken between transmission and reception is a measure of distance. This allows a picture of internal structure to be built up. In an M-mode echocardiogram the transmitter remains static, and the trace shows changes in reflections with time. In 2D echocardiograms the transmitter scans backwards and forwards, so that a two-dimensional picture is built up.

Sound reflected back from a moving target shows a shift in frequency, e.g. if the target is moving towards the source, the frequency is increased. This **Doppler** effect can be used to calculate the *velocity* of blood movement from the frequency shift in the ultrasound pulse caused by reflection from red cells. Bloodflow can then be calculated if the cross-sectional area of the vessel is estimated using echocardiography.

Cardiac catheterization and angiography

Radiopaque catheters (opaque to X-rays) are introduced into the heart or blood vessels via peripheral veins or arteries. Catheters with small balloons at the tip (**Swan–Ganz** catheters) assist placement from the venous side as the tip moves with the flow. Placement can be ascertained from the pressure waveform, and X-rays. Catheters are used for measurement of pressures or cardiac output, **angiography**, or to take samples for estimating metabolites and Po_2. Left atrial pressure cannot be measured directly, as it requires access via the mitral valve. Instead, a Swan–Ganz catheter is passed through the right heart, and wedged in a distal pulmonary artery (Fig. 32.1b). As there is thus no flow through that artery, the pressure is the same throughout the capillaries to the pulmonary vein. This **pulmonary wedge pressure** is an estimate of left atrial pressure.

Angiography

A catheter is used to introduce a radiopaque **contrast medium** into the cardiac chambers or coronary arteries. This allows visualization of the blood and vessels with X-rays, and is useful for locating blockages of the coronary circulation.

Measurement of cardiac output

All the most accurate methods for the measurement of cardiac output are invasive. These are based on **Fick's principle**, or **indicator dilution** methods.

Fick's principle

If an organ produces or takes up a substance at a constant rate, its bloodflow can be calculated from the difference between the arterial and venous concentrations, and its rate of production or uptake. This is known as **Fick's principle**. The **direct Fick method** for the estimation of cardiac output is based on the rate of O_2 consumption, and the O_2 content of the arterial and venous blood. For example, if the O_2 content of a patient's arterial blood is 190 ml O_2 per litre, and that of mixed venous blood entering the lungs is 130 ml per litre, the difference between the two (**A – V difference**) is calculated to be 60 ml per litre. This difference must have come from the lungs. If O_2 consumption is 300 ml/min, then cardiac output is:

$$CO = \frac{O_2 \text{ consumption (300 ml/min)}}{A - V \text{ difference in } O_2 \text{ content (60 ml/L)}} = 5 \text{ L/min}$$

Indicator dilution and thermodilution

If a known amount (grams) of substance is dissolved in an unknown volume of fluid, the volume can be calculated from the final concentration (gram/litre) of the substance. In **Hamilton's dye method** a quantity of nontoxic dye is injected into a vein. As it passes through the heart and lungs, it mixes with the blood, and the mean concentration is measured by taking successive arterial blood samples. A typical plot of arterial concentration vs time for rest and exercise is shown in Fig. 32.1(c). The second rise in concentration is caused by recirculation. Cardiac output is calculated from:

$$CO = \frac{\text{amount of dye injected}}{\text{mean dye concentration} \times \text{duration of first passage}}$$

A highly accurate version of this method uses lithium as the indicator, and an ion-selective electrode.

Thermodilution

In this variant cold saline is used as the indicator. It is the most commonly used method for the measurement of cardiac output. A modified Swan–Ganz catheter, with a thermistor at its tip and an opening from the lumen a few centimetres from the tip, is placed so that the tip is in the pulmonary artery and the opening is in the right atrium (Fig. 32.1d). A small amount of ice-cold saline is injected into the atrium and mixes with the blood as it passes through the ventricle. The fall in temperature of the blood as it reaches the pulmonary artery is measured by the thermistor, and is inversely proportional to the amount the cold solution is diluted, i.e. the bloodflow. Cardiac output is calculated from the amount and temperature of solution injected, the average fall in temperature at the pulmonary artery, and the time taken for the colder blood to pass the thermistor.

33 Hyperlipidaemias

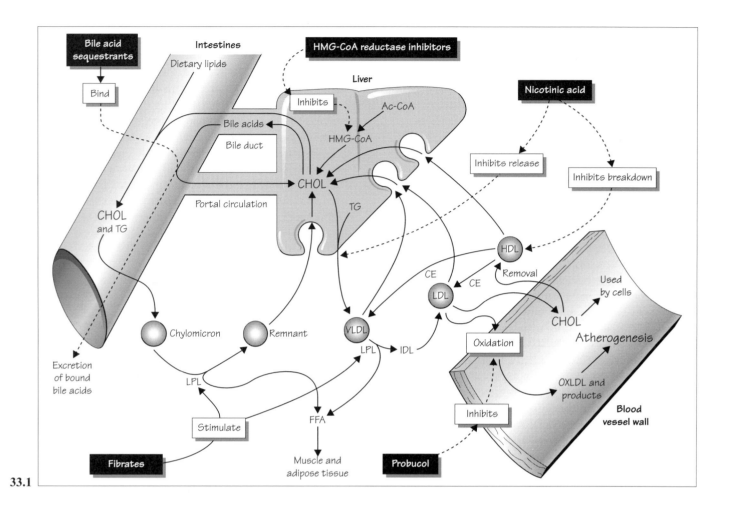

33.1

All cells require **lipids** (fats) to synthesize membranes and provide energy. Lipids are transported in the blood as **lipoproteins**. These small particles consist of a core of **triglycerides** and **cholesteryl esters**, surrounded by a coat of **phospholipids**, **cholesterol**, and proteins, termed **apolipoproteins** or **apoproteins**. Apoproteins stabilize the lipoprotein particles and help target specific types of lipoproteins to various tissues. **Hyperlipidaemias** are abnormalities of lipoprotein levels, which promote the development of *atherosclerosis* (Chapter 34) and *coronary heart disease* (CHD) (Chapters 37–39).

Lipoproteins and lipid transport

The figure illustrates pathways of lipid transport in the body. The **exogenous** pathway (left side of the figure) delivers ingested lipids to the body tissues and liver. Ingested triglycerides and cholesterol are combined with apoproteins in the intestinal mucosa to form **chylomicrons**. Passing into the bloodstream via the lymphatic system, chylomicrons bind to the capillary endothelium in muscle and adipose tissue. Here, their triglycer-

ides are hydrolysed by the enzyme **lipoprotein lipase** (LPL), yielding fatty acids which enter the tissues. The liver takes up the residual **chylomicron remnants**. These are broken down to yield cholesterol, which the liver also synthesizes. The rate-limiting enzyme in cholesterol synthesis is **hydroxymethylglutaryl coenzyme A reductase** (HMG-CoA reductase). The liver uses cholesterol to make bile acids and membrane components.

The **endogenous** pathway cycles lipids between the liver and peripheral tissues. The liver forms **very low density lipoproteins** (VLDL), consisting mainly of triglycerides, with some cholesterol. VLDL triglycerides are hydrolysed by LPL, providing fatty acids to body tissues. As it is progressively drained of triglycerides, VLDL becomes **intermediate density lipoprotein** (IDL) and then **low density lipoprotein** (LDL), losing all of its apoproteins except for **apo B100** in the process. Most of the LDL, which contains mainly cholesteryl esters, is taken up by the liver. The remaining LDL serves to distribute cholesterol to the peripheral tissues. Cells regulate their cholesterol uptake by expressing more *LDL receptors* (which bind LDL via its apo B100) when their cholesterol requirement increases.

Cholesterol is removed from tissues by **high density lipoprotein** (HDL), which is initially assembled in the plasma from lipids and apoproteins (particularly **apo A1**) lost by other lipoproteins. It accumulates cholesterol from cell membranes and transfers it (as cholesterol esters) to VLDL, IDL, and LDL, which return it to the liver.

Hyperlipidaemias: types and treatments

Primary hyperlipidaemias are caused by genetic abnormalities affecting apoproteins, apoprotein receptors, or enzymes involved in lipoprotein metabolism. *Secondary* hyperlipidaemias are caused by conditions or drugs (e.g. diabetes, renal disease, alcohol abuse, thiazide diuretics) affecting lipoprotein metabolism. Diets high in saturated fats also cause hypercholesterolaemia, probably by decreasing hepatic lipoprotein clearance. The **Frederickson/WHO classification** identifies six hyperlipidaemic phenotypes. Type IIa involves **hypercholesterolaemia** with elevated LDL-cholesterol but normal triglycerides. Types I, IV and V involve mainly **hypertriglyceridaemia**, in which VLDL and/or chylomicron levels are raised. In **hypercholesterolaemia with hypertriglyceridaemia** (types IIb and III) both cholesterol and triglycerides are elevated.

The treatment of hyperlipidaemias aims to lower LDL-cholesterol and/or triglycerides, and to raise HDL-cholesterol. Patients with CHD or multiple cardiovascular risk factors require an especially aggressive normalization of lipid levels. Therapy reduces the risk of CHD, and can cause the *regression* of existing atherosclerotic lesions. Desirable total and LDL serum cholesterol levels are less than 200 mg/dl (5.2 mmol/L) and 130 mg/dl (3.4 mmol/L), respectively. The National Cholesterol Education Program in the United States suggests that lipid-lowering therapy should be considered in those free of overt CHD if their serum LDL-cholesterol is above 130 mg/dl (3.4 mmol/L) if two or more other risk factors are present, and when LDL-cholesterol is above 160 mg/dl (4.1 mmol/L) with one coexisting risk factor. For patients with CHD, therapy is recommended if LDL-cholesterol is more than 100 mg/dl (2.6 mmol/L). Treatment often begins with a low-fat, high carbohydrate diet. If this fails to normalize hyperlipidaemia adequately after 6 months, therapy with a lipid-lowering drug is considered.

HMG-CoA reductase inhibitors or 'statins' include **simvastatin, lovastatin, pravastatin, fluvastatin, mevastatin,** and **atorvastatin**. The West of Scotland Coronary Prevention Study (WOSCOPS) reported in 1995 that treatment of middle-aged men with high cholesterol but no history of myocardial infarction (MI) using pravastatin reduced the incidence of MI or death from cardiovascular disease by 31% over a 5-year period. Remarkably, the AFCAPS/TexCAPS trial reported in 1998 that over a similar period lovastatin reduced the incidence of first MI by 40% in individuals with low HDL but *average*

cholesterol levels. Statins reduce hepatic synthesis of cholesterol, causing an upregulation of hepatic receptors for B and E apoproteins. This increases the clearance of LDL, IDL and VLDL from the plasma. Statins also increase plasma HDL levels by an unknown mechanism. These drugs are most appropriate for patients with overt CHD or pronounced hypercholesterolaemia. Serious adverse effects associated with their use are very rare. They include *hepatoxicity* and *rhabdomyolysis* (destruction of skeletal muscle), the risk of which is increased with concomitant use of nicotinic acid or a fibric acid derivative.

Bile acid sequestrants: Bile acids are synthesized from cholesterol in the liver, and cycle between the liver and intestine (enterohepatic recirculation). **Cholestyramine** and **cholestipol** are exchange resins that bind and trap bile acids in the intestine, increasing their excretion. This enhances hepatic bile acid synthesis and cholesterol utilization. The resulting depletion of hepatic cholesterol causes an upregulation of LDL receptors, increasing the clearance of LDL-cholesterol from the plasma. The bile acid sequestrants cause little systemic toxicity because they are not absorbed. They are, however, taken in large amounts (e.g. up to 30 g/day), and cause gastrointestinal side effects such as nausea, diarrhoea, and reflux oesophagitis.

Nicotinic acid is a B vitamin that has lipid-lowering effects at high doses. It inhibits the synthesis and release of VLDL by the liver. Because VLDL gives rise to IDL and LDL, plasma levels of these lipoproteins also fall. Conversely, HDL levels rise as a result of decreased breakdown. Nicotinic acid can cause a number of adverse effects, including hepatotoxicity, palpitations, impairment of glucose tolerance, hyperuricaemia, hypotension, and amblyopia. Most patients experience flushing when starting nicotinic acid therapy. This is caused by vasodilatation, which is secondary to prostaglandin release from the endothelium. This can be prevented by nonsteroidal anti-inflammatory drugs.

Fibric acid deriviatives (fibrates) include **gemfibrazole, clofibrate, bezafibrate, ciprofibrate,** and **fenofibrate**. These stimulate the activity of lipoprotein lipase, thereby reducing VLDL triglycerides by increasing their hydrolysis. They also promote changes in LDL composition, which render it less atherogenic, and enhance fibrolysis. Fibrates are mainly used with types IIb and III hyperlipidaemias. They cause mild gastrointestinal disorders in 5–10% of patients, and can potentially cause muscle toxicity and renal failure if combined with HMG-CoA reductase inhibitors or excessive alcohol use.

Probucol is an antioxidant that is similar in structure to the preservative BHT. It lowers both LDL-cholesterol and HDL-cholesterol by unknown mechanisms, but its efficacy in retarding atherosclerosis progression is probably caused by an inhibition of LDL oxidation. It may cause cardiac arrhythmias. **Oestrogen** reduces LDL-cholesterol and increases HDL-cholesterol. It reduces CHD risk by 40–50% when given to postmenopausal women, and is usually combined with progesterone, which reduces its tendency to cause endometrial cancer.

34 Atherosclerosis

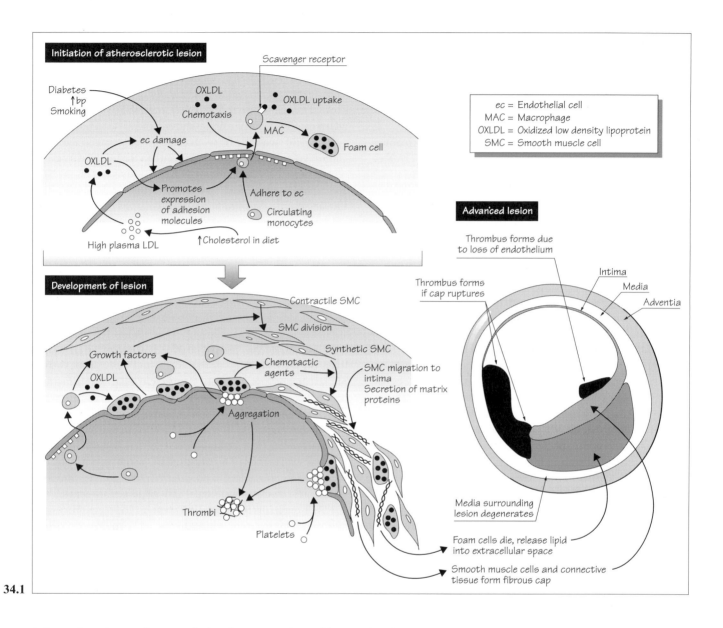

34.1

Atherosclerosis, a disease of the larger arteries, ultimately causes almost 50% of mortality in the Western world. Atherosclerosis begins in childhood with **fatty streaks**, localized accumulations of lipid within the arterial intima. By middle age some of these develop into **atherosclerotic plaques**, focal lesions where the arterial wall is grossly abnormal. Plaques may be several centimetres across, and are most common in the *aorta*, the *coronary* and *internal carotid arteries*, and the *circle of Willis*. An advanced atherosclerotic plaque, illustrated on the right of the diagram, demonstrates several features.

1 The arterial wall is focally thickened by intimal smooth muscle cell proliferation and the deposition of fibrous connective tissue, forming a hard **fibrous cap**. This projects into the vascular lumen, restricting the flow of blood, and often causes ischaemia in the tissue region served by the artery.

2 A soft pool of extracellular lipid and cell debris accumulates beneath the fibrous cap (*athera* is Greek for gruel or porridge). This weakens the arterial wall, so that the fibrous cap may fissure or tear away. As a result, blood enters the lesions and **thrombi** (blood clots) are formed. These thrombi, or the material leaking from the ruptured lesion, may be carried to the upstream vascular bed to *embolize* (plug) smaller vessels. A larger thrombus may totally occlude (block) the artery at the site of the lesion. This causes myocardial infarction or stroke if it occurs in a coronary or cerebral artery, respectively.

3 The endothelium over the lesion is partially or completely lost. This can lead to ongoing formation of thrombi, causing intermittent flow occlusion as in unstable angina.

4 The medial smooth muscle layer under the lesion degenerates. This weakens the vascular wall, which may distend and eventually rupture (an **aneurysm**). Aneurysms are especially common in the abdominal aorta.

Atherosclerotic arteries may also demonstrate spasms or reduced vasodilatation. This worsens the restriction of the bloodflow and promotes thrombus formation (Chapters 37–39).

Pathogenesis of atherosclerosis

The risk of developing atherosclerosis is in part genetically determined. The incidence of clinical consequences of atherosclerosis such as ischaemic heart disease rises with age, especially after age 40. Atherosclerosis is much more common in men than in women. This difference is probably due to a protective effect of oestrogen, and progressively disappears after menopause. Important risk factors that predispose towards atherosclerosis include smoking, hypertension, diabetes and high serum cholesterol.

The most widely accepted hypothesis for the pathogenesis of atherosclerosis proposes that it is initiated by *endothelial injury or dysfunction*. Plaques tend to develop in areas of variable haemodynamic sheer stress (e.g. where arteries branch or bifurcate). The endothelium is especially vulnerable to damage at such sites, as evidenced by increased endothelial cell turnover and permeability. Endothelial dysfunction promotes the adhesion of **monocytes**, white blood cells which burrow beneath the endothelial monolayer and become **macrophages**. Macrophages normally play an important role during inflammation, the body's response to injury and infection. They do so by acting as scavenger cells to remove dead cells and foreign material, and also by subsequently releasing *cytokines* and *growth factors* to promote healing. As described below, however, macrophages in the arterial wall can be abnormally activated, causing a type of slow inflammatory reaction, which eventually results in advanced and clinically dangerous plaques.

Oxidized low density lipoprotein, macrophages, and atherogenesis

Lipoproteins transport cholesterol and other lipids in the bloodstream (see Chapter 33). Elevated levels of one type of lipoprotein, low density lipoprotein (LDL), are associated with atherosclerosis. Native LDL is not atherogenic. However, oxidative modification of LDL by oxidants derived from macrophages and endothelial and smooth muscle cells can lead to the generation of highly atherogenic **oxidized LDL** within the vascular wall.

Oxidized LDL is thought to promote atherogenesis through several mechanisms (see upper panel of Fig. 34.1). Oxidized LDL is chemotactic for (i.e. attracts) circulating monocytes, and increases the expression of endothelial cell adhesion molecules to which monocytes attach. The monocytes then penetrate the endothelial monolayer, lodge beneath it, and mature into macrophages. Cellular uptake of native LDL is normally highly regulated. However, certain cells, including macrophages, are unable to control their uptake of oxidized LDL, which occurs via **scavenger receptors**. Once within the vascular wall, macrophages therefore accumulate large quantities of oxidized LDL, eventually becoming the cholesterol-laden **foam cells** forming the fatty streak.

As shown in the lower left of the figure, stimulation of macrophages and endothelial cells by oxidized LDL then causes these cells to release cytokines. T lymphocytes may also enter the vascular wall and release cytokines. Additional cytokines are released by platelets aggregating on the endothelium at the site at which it has been damaged by oxidized LDL and other toxic substances released by the foam cells. The cytokines act on the vascular smooth muscle cells of the media, causing them to *migrate into the intima, to proliferate*, and to *secrete abnormal amounts of collagen and other connective tissue proteins*. Over time, the intimal accumulation of smooth muscle cells and connective tissue forms the fibrous cap on the inner arterial wall. Underneath this, ongoing foam cell formation and deterioration forms a layer of extracellular lipid (largely cholesterol and cholesteryl esters) and cellular debris. Still-viable foam cells often localize at the edges or shoulders of the lesion. Underneath the lipid, the medial layer of smooth muscle cells is weakened and atrophied.

Clinical consequences of advanced atherosclerosis

Atherosclerotic lesions are of most clinical consequence when they occur in the coronary arteries. As the fibrous cap thickens, it may cause a **stenosis**, or narrowing of the vascular lumen. When stenosis reaches approximately 70%, the flow of blood becomes sufficiently restricted to cause ischaemia when myocardial oxygen demand rises. This leads to **stable** or **exertional angina** (see Chapter 37). Advanced plaques often have large areas of endothelial denudation, which serve as sites for thrombus formation. In addition, lipid- and foam-cell-rich lesions are particularly unstable and prone to tearing open. The formation of fissures allows blood to enter the lesion, causing thrombi to form on the surface and/or within the lesion. This can lead to such consequences as:

1 Increased stenosis as the lesion is expanded.

2 Plugging of smaller downstream vessels by thrombi released from the lesion.

3 Partial or complete occlusion of the artery by a thrombus at the lesion itself.

Depending on the location and extent of the occluded artery, **unstable angina** (see Chapter 38) or **myocardial infarction** (see Chapter 40) may occur. Non-fatal chronic thrombi may gradually be replaced by connective tissue and incorporated into the lesion, a process termed **organization**.

Atherosclerosis of cerebral arteries is the major cause of **stroke** (cerebral infarction). Atherosclerotic stenosis of the renal arteries causes about two-thirds of cases of **renovascular hypertension**.

35 Diagnosis and treatment of hypertension

Table 35.1 JNC-V classification of adult blood pressure.

Classification	Systolic (mmHg)		Diastolic (mmHg)
Normotension	< 130	and/or	< 85
High normal	130–139	and/or	85–89
Stage 1 (mild) HT	140–159	and/or	90–99
Stage 2 (moderate) HT	160–179	and/or	100–109
Stage 3 (severe) HT	180–209	and/or	110–119
Stage 4 (very severe) HT	210	and/or	120

The risk of developing cardiovascular disease increases progressively with *both* systolic and diastolic blood pressure levels. **Hypertension** is defined pragmatically as the level of blood pressure above which therapeutic intervention can be shown to reduce risk. Table 35.1 shows the blood pressure classification system proposed in 1994 by the Fifth Report of the Joint National Committee on Detection, Evaluation, and Treatment of High Blood Pressure (JNC-V) in the USA. Blood pressure measurements can vary significantly, necessitating confirmation of all but severe hypertension by repeated measurements made over at least two separate occasions.

As Table 35.1 shows, an elevation of either the diastolic and/or systolic blood pressure constitutes hypertension. The deleterious effects of **isolated systolic hypertension** (ISH) are increasingly recognized.

Treatment of hypertension

Epidemiological studies predict that a long-term 5–6 mmHg diminution of diastolic blood pressure (DBP) should reduce the incidence of stroke and CHD by about 40% and 25%, respectively. Clinical trials (mainly using β-blockers and diuretics) show that pharmacological reduction of DBP by this amount for 5 years reduces stroke incidence by the predicted amount, however CHD is reduced by only 15–20%. These studies demonstrate that antihypertensive treatment greatly decreases cardiovascular mortality, but suggest that further therapeutic improvements are possible.

Controversy exists as to the level of blood pressure at which the benefits of treatment with drugs outweigh costs and possible adverse effects. A recent report by the World Health Organization recommends considering drug treatment when the DBP remains between 95 and 105 mmHg for more than 6 months, or if the DBP remains between 90 and 95 mmHg if certain cardiovascular risk factors are present. Relevant risk factors include *overt cardiovascular disease, diabetes, obesity, dyslipidaemia,* a *family history of cardiovascular disease,* or *disease of target organs* vulnerable to hypertension (e.g. kidneys and brain). There is an emerging consensus that mild hypertension should be treated if a patient's overall risk of cardiovascular events (e.g. MI), as estimated using risk tables derived from the Framingham

study (see Chapter 31), exceeds 2% per year. The goal of antihypertensive therapy is to reduce the blood pressure to below 140/90 mmHg.

There is abundant evidence that **lifestyle modifications** such as *weight reduction, regular aerobic exercise,* and *limitation of dietary sodium* and *alcohol intake* can often normalize pressure in mild hypertensives. They are also useful adjuncts to pharmacological therapy of more severe disease, and have the important added bonus of reducing overall cardiovascular risk.

Antihypertensive drugs act to reduce cardiac output and/or total peripheral resistance. The major classes of antihypertensive drugs include β**-adrenoceptor blockers, diuretics, angiotensin-converting enzyme inhibitors (ACEI), Ca²⁺-channel antagonists,** and α_1**-receptor blockers** (Table 35.2). Therapy is usually initiated with a drug from one of these classes. At present, β-blockers and diuretics are usually recommended as initial drugs for uncomplicated hypertension because these have been shown by clinical trials to reduce mortality. However, as other types of antihypertensive drugs can often exert beneficial actions on coexisting conditions (e.g. ACEI on heart failure), these drugs may be more appropriate for many patients (Table 35.2). Inadequate or adverse responses to the first drug tried necessitate substitution with an agent from another class. In some cases combinations of two or three drugs are needed.

Diuretics can be used with vasodilators (e.g. α_1-blockers, Ca^{2+}-channel antagonists), which may elicit volume expansion and oedema due to RAA system activation. Diuretics cause hypokalaemia by promoting Na^+/K^+ exchange in the collecting tubule (see Chapter 44). This can be prevented by also giving K^+-sparing diuretics (e.g. amiloride) to reduce Na^+ reabsorption by blocking Na^+ channels in the collecting duct.

α_1**-receptor-selective blockers** are used in preference to nonselective α-antagonists in order to prevent the increased norepinephrine release from sympathetic nerves, which would occur if presynaptic α_2-receptors were also blocked.

It has recently been proposed that **Ca²⁺-channel antagonists,** particularly those which are short acting, may increase mortality via pro-ischaemic and other effects. Conversely, the Sys-Eur Trial reported in 1997 that long-acting nitrendipine reduced stroke incidence in elderly patients with ISH. It is presently recommended that short-acting dihydropyridines should not be prescribed, although other Ca^{2+} antagonists may be used when indicated. Large trials examining the safety and efficacy of Ca^{2+} antagonists are in progress.

A variety of other drugs are effective in reducing blood pressure, but are used less widely. The older centrally acting drugs **clonidine**, **guanabenz**, and **guanfacine** inhibit sympathetic outflow by stimulating α_2-receptors in the medulla. α**-methyl dopa** has a similar effect after being converted in the brain to α-methyl norepinephrine, and is the drug of choice for the

Table 35.2 Major classes of antihypertensive drugs.

Class	Drugs	Adverse effects	Indications (I)/ Contraindications (C)	Mechanisms
Thiazide diuretics Thiazide-related diuretics	Bendroflumathazide Benzthiazide Chlorothiazide Hydrochlorothiazide Hydroflumethiazide Chlortalidone Indapamide Xipamide Metolazone	Hypokalaemia, increased plasma insulin, glucose, cholesterol, hypersensitivity reactions, impotence	(I): old age, black race congestive heart failure (C): dyslipidaemia	Initial increased Na^+ excretion by kidneys causes fall in blood volume and cardiac output. This is due to inhibition of Na^+/Cl^- symport in distal nephron. Subsequently, blood volume recovers, but total peripheral resistance falls due to unknown mechanism (possibly opening of ATP-dependent K^+ channels in vascular smooth muscle cells)
β-receptor blockers NS = blocks $β_1$ and $β_2$ S = $β_1$ selective PβA = partial β-receptor agonist α = also blocks α-receptors	Propranolol (NS) Nadolol (NS) Timolol (NS) Pindolol (NS, PβA) Atenolol (S) Metoprolol (S) Acebutolol (S, PβA) Celiprolol (S, PβA) Labetalol (α) Bucindolol (α) Carvidelol (α)	Bronchospasm, fatigue, negative inotropy, CNS disturbances with some (e.g. nightmares), worsening and masking signs of hypoglycaemia, dyslipidaemia (less if PβA)	(I): angina, after myocardial infarction (C): asthma, diabetes, peripheral vascular disease, dyslipidaemia	Reduce cardiac output via negative inotropic and chronotropic effect. This is mediated by blockade of cardiac β receptors (mainly $β_1$). stimulated by the sympathetic nervous system. Also, inhibition of renin release by blockade of β receptors on juxtaglomerular granule cells. Total peripheral resistance rises initially and then returns to pre-drug level via an unknown mechanism
α-receptor blockers	Prazosin Terazosin Doxazosin	Postural hypotension, esp. on first dosing, oedema (give with a diuretic). Also, less commonly: fatigue, dizziness, urinary incontinence	(I): diabetes, dyslipidaemia, benign prostatic hypertrophy	Reduce total peripheral resistance by blocking sympathetic activation of vascular $α_1$ adrenoceptors. Dilates arteries and veins, with little effect on cardiac output. May increase insulin sensitivity and improve plasma lipid profile
Ca²⁺-channel blockers	Nifedipine Amlodipine Nicardipine Isradipine Felodipine Lacidipine Diltiazem Verapamil	Headache, flushing, fatigue, tachycardia, peripheral oedema. Bradycardia, negative inotropy, SA and AV node block with verapamil and diltiazem	(I): angina, renal insufficiency, cerebrovascular disease (C): congestive heart failure, pregnancy. Avoid combination with β-blockers	Reduce total peripheral resistance by dilating resistance arteries. The drugs promote the inactivation of voltage-gated Ca^{2+} channels in vascular smooth muscle cells; this inhibits Ca^{2+} influx and therefore force development. Verapamil and diltiazem also have a significant effect on cardiac Ca^{2+} channels
ACE inhibitors	Captopril Enalopril Lisinopril Benazepril Fosinopril Ramipril Quinapril Perindopril Trandolipril	First dose postural hypotension, cough, acute renal failure, fatigue, headache, dizziness, allergic reactions	(I): congestive heart failure, postmyocardial infarction, diabetes (C): pregnancy, renovascular disease, aortic stenosis	Block the conversion of angiotensin I into angiotensin II. This reduces total peripheral resistance because angiotensin II stimulates the sympathetic system centrally, promotes release of norepinephrine from sympathetic nerves, and vasoconstricts directly. Also promotes diuresis/natriuresis

treatment of chronic hypertension in pregnancy. These agents cause sedation. The newer agents **rilmenidine** and **moxonidine** reduce sympathetic outflow by activating central *imidazoline* (I_1) receptors; this lowers blood pressure, possibly with less sedation than that caused by $α_2$-agonists. **Minoxidil** is a powerful vasodilator used in refractory hypertension. It opens ATP-sensitive K^+ channels in vascular smooth muscle cells, causing a hyperpolarization which closes Ca^{2+} channels. Oedema and

tachycardia are adverse effects that can be controlled by coadministering a β-blocker and diuretic. Angiotensin II receptor antagonists, such as **losartan** and **valsartan**, have also recently been introduced. These may be used in patients who cannot tolerate ACEI because of persistent coughing.

In cases in which hypertension is secondary to a known condition or factor (e.g. renal stenosis, oral contraceptives), removal of this cause is often sufficient to normalize the blood pressure.

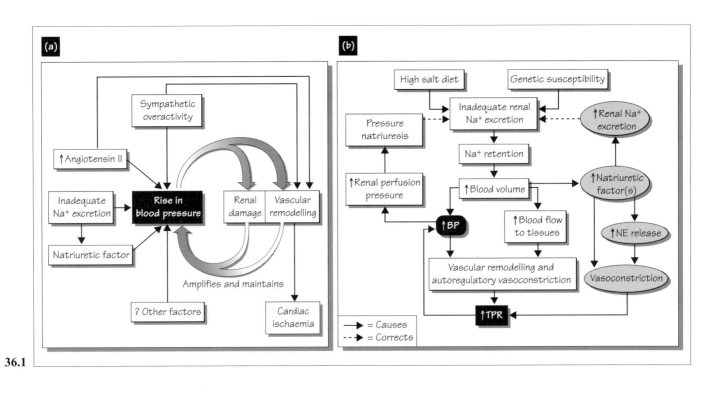

In > 90% of cases, hypertension has no obvious cause, and is termed **primary** or **essential**. Primary hypertension is a **multifactorial genetic disorder**, in which inheritance of a number of abnormal genes predisposes an individual to high blood pressure, especially if appropriate **environmental influences** (e.g. high salt diet, psychosocial stress) are also present. The identities of the genes involved are presently unresolved, and attempts to define causative mechanisms have mainly focused on uncovering functional abnormalities associated with hypertension. This approach has been aided by the development through selective breeding programmes of hypertensive strains of animals, such as the spontaneously hypertensive rat (SHR) and the Milan hypertensive rat. It is hoped that some of the mechanisms causing hypertension are similar enough across species that their elucidation in animals will provide important clues to the human disease.

Studies tracking cardiovascular function over many years have shown that early human hypertension is often associated with an increased cardiac output (CO) and heart rate, but a normal total peripheral resistance (TPR). Over a period of years, CO falls to subnormal levels, while TPR becomes permanently increased, thereby maintaining the hypertension (recall that blood pressure = CO × TPR). One important implication of these and other studies is that the factors maintaining the elevated blood pressure may change over a period of time. Many authorities therefore feel that high blood pressure can be initiated by a variety of factors (e.g. insufficient Na+ excretion, sympathetic overactivity), but is then amplified and maintained

mainly by common secondary mechanisms such as renal damage and vascular structural remodelling which are caused by the initial rise in pressure. This unifying hypothesis for primary hypertension is shown in Fig. 36.1(a).

The kidney and sodium in hypertension

As described in Chapter 28, the kidneys regulate long-term blood pressure by controlling the body's Na+ content. It has been proposed that primary hypertension is caused by renal abnormalities which cause *impaired* or *inadequate Na+ excretion* (Fig. 36.1a). According to this model, the resulting Na+ retention increases blood volume and CO. These changes then promote Na+ excretion by causing pressure natriuresis (see Chapter 28). Fluid balance is restored, but at the cost of a rise in blood pressure. Over the long term, the rise in blood pressure or flow would set in train *autoregulatory* processes resulting in vasoconstriction and/or vascular structural remodelling. This would reduce blood volume to normal levels, but by raising TPR would maintain the high blood pressure needed for Na+ balance.

Extensive evidence suggests that this renal mechanism of primary hypertension may be important in many individuals. For example, a high salt diet, which should exacerbate the renal deficiency in Na+ excretion, worsens hypertension in many patients and raises blood pressure in some normotensives. In addition, it has been shown that blood pressure falls when the kidneys from normotensives are transplanted into hypertensives. More recently, impairment of renal Na+ excretion has been demonstrated directly in **Liddle syndrome**, a rare form of human hypertension in which a mutation of the mineralocorticoid-sensitive Na^+ channel causes its continual overactivity.

The natriuretic factor hypothesis

An extension of the renal hypothesis (right side of Fig. 36.1a) proposes that the body responds to inadequate renal salt excretion by producing one or more **natriuretic factors** (not to be confused with **atrial natriuretic peptide**, see Chapter 28) that promote salt excretion by inhibiting the Na^+ pumps in the nephron. Na^+ pumps are also indirectly involved in lowering intracellular Ca^{2+}, via regulation of both the membrane potential and Na^+/Ca^{2+} exchange in smooth muscle cells and neurones. Natriuretic factors would therefore cause additional responses such as vasoconstriction, increased norepinephrine release, and possibly stimulation of brain centres involved in raising blood pressure. These effects would increase TPR, causing sustained hypertension. In agreement with this hypothesis, several endogenous substances that inhibit the Na^+ pump, one being almost identical in structure to ouabain, have been found to be elevated in the plasma from hypertensives.

The renin–angiotensin–aldosterone (RAA) system in hypertension

Although renin release should be greatly suppressed by elevated blood pressure, many hypertensives have normal or even high plasma renin activity. It has been proposed that this is caused by an abnormality of renin release which would lead both to angiotensin II-mediated vasoconstriction and to Na^+ retention via aldosterone, both mechanisms causing hypertension. Angiotensin II is also a potent stimulator of the sympathetic nervous system. Primary hypertension in some individuals has also been linked to a mutation in the **angiotensinogen** gene, which could promote increased angiotensin II production.

Neurogenic hypertension

The neurogenic model of hypertension suggests that blood pressure elevation is primarily initiated by defective neurohumoral regulation of blood pressure. Supporters of this concept stress that the central nervous system is ultimately the final determinant of blood pressure, because it can exert long-term influences on renal function (e.g. bloodflow), on the production of vasoactive substances, and on vascular and cardiac structure. The neurogenic model is supported by evidence that sympathetic nervous activity is increased in young borderline hypertensives, and also by the finding that the SHR can be permanently 'cured' if its (overactive) sympathetic nervous system is rendered ineffective soon after birth. It may also explain studies in which 'stress' has been linked to hypertension. A recent report suggests that the venous circulation in hypertensives is unusually sensitive to the endothelium-derived vasoconstrictor **endothelin**.

Vascular remodelling

Established hypertension is associated with the *structural alteration* of small arteries and larger arterioles. This process, termed **remodelling**, results in the narrowing of these vessels and an increase in the ratio of the wall thickness to the lumenal radius. These changes are thought to constitute an adaptive response to a rise in blood pressure to protect the microcirculation from the increased blood pressure. Remodelling may also be enhanced by the RAA and sympathetic nervous systems, the activation of which are known to promote smooth muscle cell growth.

Remodelling will increase basal TPR and also exaggerate the increase in TPR caused by vasoconstriction. This implies that remodelling would accentuate increases in blood pressure caused by other factors, thereby leading to the vicious cycle illustrated in Fig. 36.1(a). In addition, remodelling of the coronary arteries as a result of hypertension may increase the risk of myocardial infarction by restricting the ability of these vessels to increase the cardiac blood supply during ischaemia. It should be noted, however, that the role of remodelling in hypertension is, like much else in this area of research, the subject of intense ongoing controversy.

Secondary hypertension

In <10% of cases, high blood pressure can be traced to a known condition or factor. Common causes of such **secondary hypertension** include:

1 *Renal parenchymal* and *renovascular diseases* which impair volume regulation and/or activate the renin–angiotensin–aldosterone system.

2 *Endocrine disturbances*, often of the adrenal cortex, and associated with the oversecretion of aldosterone, cortisol, and/or catecholamines.

3 *Oral contraceptives*, which may raise blood pressure via RAA activation and hyperinsulinaemia.

Malignant or accelerated hypertension is an uncommon condition which develops quickly, involves large elevations in pressure, is often secondary to other conditions, rapidly damages the kidneys, retina, brain, and heart, and if untreated causes death within 1–2 years.

Consequences of hypertension

Chronic hypertension causes changes in arteries similar to those due to ageing. These include endothelial damage and **arteriosclerosis**, a thickening and increased connective tissue content of the arterial wall that causes reduced arterial compliance. These effects on vascular structure combine with elevated arterial pressure to promote atherosclerosis, coronary heart disease (CHD), left ventricular hypertrophy, and renal damage. Hypertension is therefore an important risk factor for *myocardial infarction (MI), congestive heart failure, stroke,* and *renal failure*. Almost all untreated hypertensives die from one of these conditions.

37 Stable and variant angina

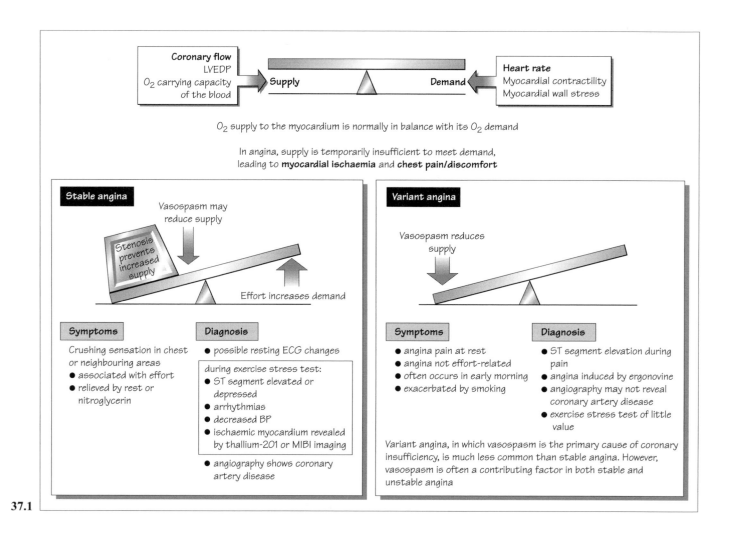

Angina pectoris is an episodic pain or crushing/squeezing sensation in the chest caused by reversible myocardial ischaemia. The discomfort may radiate into the neck, jaw, arms (particularly the left) and, more rarely, into the back. Other common symptoms include shortness of breath, abdominal pain, dizziness. Syncope (collapse) occurs infrequently. Ischaemia may produce classic angina or may be totally **silent** without any symptoms. The clinical outlook from silent ischaemia is similar to symptomatic angina.

Three forms of angina are recognized. **Stable** and **variant** angina are discussed below, and **unstable angina** is described in Chapter 38.

Pathophysiology

The figure shows the factors that determine myocardial O_2 supply and demand. O_2 demand is determined by **heart rate**, **left ventricular contractility**, and **systolic wall stress**, and therefore increases with **exercise**, **hypertension**, and **left ventricular**

dilatation (e.g. during chronic heart failure). Myocardial O_2 supply is primarily determined by coronary bloodflow and coronary vascular resistance, which mostly occurs at the level of the intramyocardial arterioles. With exercise the coronary bloodflow can increase to four to six times baseline, which is normal coronary flow reserve (see Chapter 24).

Stable or **exertional/typical** angina arises when the flow reserve of one or more coronary arteries is limited by a significant structural stenosis (> 70%) resulting from atherosclerotic coronary heart disease. Stenoses typically develop in the epicardial region of arteries, within 6 cm of the aorta. Under resting conditions, cardiac O_2 demand is low enough to be satisfied even by a diminished coronary flow. When, however, exertion or emotional stress increases myocardial O_2 demand, dilatation of the nondiseased areas of the artery is unable to increase the supply of blood to the heart because stenosis presents a fixed, nondilating obstruction. The resulting imbalance between myocardial O_2 demand and supply causes myocardial ischaemia.

Ischaemia develops mainly in the **subendocardium**, the inner part of the myocardial wall. As described in Chapter 24, the bloodflow to the left ventricular wall occurs mainly during diastole, as a result of arteriolar compression during systole. The arterioles of the subendocardium are compressed more than those of the mid- or subepicardial layers, so that the subendocardium is most vulnerable to a relative lack of O_2.

In addition to causing pain, ischaemia causes a decline in myocardial cell high-energy phosphates (creatine phosphate and ATP). As a result, both ventricular contractility and diastolic relaxation in the territory of affected arteries are impaired. Consequences of these events may include a fall in cardiac output, symptoms of pulmonary congestion, and activation of the sympathetic nervous system. Stable angina is almost always relieved within 5–10 min by rest or by nitroglycerin, which reduces cardiac O_2 demand.

Some patients with stable angina may have excellent effort tolerance one day, but develop angina with minimal activity on another day. Contributing to this phenomenon of *variable threshold angina* is a dynamic endothelial dysfunction that often occurs in patients with coronary artery disease. The endothelium normally acts via nitric oxide to dilate coronary arteries during exercise. If this endothelium-dependent vasodilatation is periodically impaired, exercise may result in paradoxical vasoconstriction as a result of the unopposed vasoconstricting effect of the sympathetic nervous system on coronary α receptors.

Variant angina, also termed **vasospastic** or **Prinzmetal's** angina, is an uncommon condition in which myocardial ischaemia and pain are caused by a severe transient **occlusive spasm** of one or more epicardial coronary arteries. Variant angina occurs at rest (typically in the early morning hours) and may be intensely painful. It is exacerbated by smoking, and can be precipitated by cocaine use. About 30% of these patients show no evidence of coronary atherosclerotic lesions. Vasospasm is thought to occur because a segment of artery becomes abnormally over-reactive to vasoconstricting agents (e.g. norepinephrine, serotonin).

Diagnosis

Ischaemic heart disease and stable angina can be distinguished from other conditions causing chest pain (e.g. neuromuscular disorders, gastroesophageal reflux) on the basis of characteristic anginal symptoms and several types of diagnostic investigation. Although *resting ST/T wave changes* indicate severe underlying coronary artery disease, the resting ECG is often normal. In this case, the presence of ischaemic heart disease can be unmasked by an **exercise stress test**, during which patients exercise at a progressively increasing level of effort on a stationary bicycle or treadmill. Development of cardiac ischaemia is revealed by chest pain, ECG changes including *S–T segment depression* or *elevation*, arrhythmias, or a fall in blood pressure due to reduced ventricular contractility. The degree of effort at which these signs develop indicates the severity of ischaemia.

The exercise stress test is less useful in uncovering ischaemia-related ECG changes if the baseline ECG is already abnormal as a result of factors such as left bundle branch block. In such patients, techniques designed to visualize ischaemic myocardium can be combined with the stress test to increase its specificity. **Thallium-201** is an isotope that is taken up by normal but not ischaemic or previously infarcted myocardium. It is given intravenously during the stress test, and a gamma camera is used to image its distribution in the heart both immediately and also after the test, when ischaemia has subsided. A region of exercise-induced ischaemia will cause a 'cold spot' during but not after the stress test, because it will take up thallium-201 when ischaemia has passed. **^{99m}Tc-methoxy isobutyl isonitrile (MIBI)** can also be used for this purpose. **Coronary angiography** (see Chapter 32) is used to provide direct radiographic visualization of the extent and severity of coronary artery disease, allowing risk assessment.

The hallmark of variant angina is S–T segment elevation on the ECG. Cardiac ischaemia caused by variant angina may cause ventricular arryhthmias, syncope, and even MI during prolonged attacks. Variant angina is provoked by intravenous administration of the vasoconstrictor **ergonovine**, forming the basis of a hospital test for this condition.

Prognosis
Stable angina
Mortality is 2–4% a year if only one coronary artery is diseased, but increases with the number of diseased arteries, especially if there is significant stenosis in the left coronary artery mainstem. Patients with poor left ventricular function are at particular risk.

Variant angina
Patients without significant coronary artery disease have a benign prognosis; in a recent study only 4% of patients in this group died from a cardiac cause during an average follow-up period of 7 years. However, patients who also have severe coronary artery disease or who develop severe arrhythmias during vasospastic episodes are at greater risk.

Management
The management of angina is designed to control symptoms, reduce underlying risk factors, and improve prognosis. **Drug therapy** utilizes nitrovasodilators, β-adrenoceptor blockers, Ca^{2+}-channel antagonists, and drugs that inhibit platelet aggregation and thrombosis (see Chapters 39, 42). Minimization of **risk factors** (see Chapter 31) is a vital component of treatment. Stable angina can also be treated using the **revascularization** techniques described in Chapter 38.

38 Unstable angina and revascularization

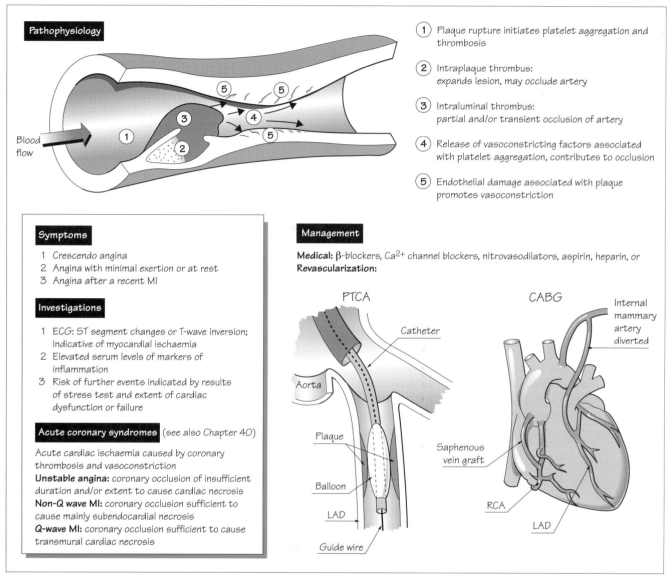

Pathophysiology

① Plaque rupture initiates platelet aggregation and thrombosis

② Intraplaque thrombus: expands lesion, may occlude artery

③ Intraluminal thrombus: partial and/or transient occlusion of artery

④ Release of vasoconstricting factors associated with platelet aggregation, contributes to occlusion

⑤ Endothelial damage associated with plaque promotes vasoconstriction

Blood flow

Symptoms

1 Crescendo angina
2 Angina with minimal exertion or at rest
3 Angina after a recent MI

Investigations

1 ECG: ST segment changes or T-wave inversion; indicative of myocardial ischaemia
2 Elevated serum levels of markers of inflammation
3 Risk of further events indicated by results of stress test and extent of cardiac dysfunction or failure

Acute coronary syndromes (see also Chapter 40)

Acute cardiac ischaemia caused by coronary thrombosis and vasoconstriction
Unstable angina: coronary occlusion of insufficient duration and/or extent to cause cardiac necrosis
Non-Q wave MI: coronary occlusion sufficient to cause mainly subendocardial necrosis
Q-wave MI: coronary occlusion sufficient to cause transmural cardiac necrosis

Management

Medical: β-blockers, Ca^{2+} channel blockers, nitrovasodilators, aspirin, heparin, or
Revascularization:

PTCA

Catheter

Aorta

Plaque

Balloon

LAD

Guide wire

CABG

Internal mammary artery diverted

Saphenous vein graft

RCA

LAD

38.1

Unstable angina is a dangerous condition, which often heralds impending myocardial infarction (MI). Unstable angina has several presentations, including:

1 Crescendo angina, where attacks are progressively more severe, prolonged, and frequent.

2 Angina of recent onset (some weeks) brought on by minimal exertion.

3 Angina occurring at rest/with minimal exertion or during sleep.

4 Post-MI angina (ischaemic pain 24 h to 2 weeks after MI).

Symptoms resemble those of stable angina, but they are frequently more intense and persistent, often lasting 30 min. Pain is frequently resistant to nitroglycerin.

Pathophysiology

Studies have shown that unstable angina episodes are preceded by a fall in coronary bloodflow. This is thought to result from the periodic development of coronary **thrombosis** and **vasoconstriction**, which are triggered by coronary artery disease.

Thrombosis is promoted by the endothelial damage and turbulent bloodflow associated with atherosclerotic plaques. Compared to the lesions of stable angina, plaques found in patients with unstable angina tend to have a thinner fibrous cap and a larger lipid core, and are generally more widespread and severe. The stenoses in unstable angina are often **eccentric**; the plaque does not surround the entire circumference of the artery. Such lesions are especially vulnerable to being **ruptured** by haemodynamic stress. This exposes the plaque interior, which powerfully stimulates platelet aggregation and thrombosis. The thrombus propagates out into the coronary lumen, partially occluding the artery. Rupture may also cause haemorrhage into the lesion itself, expanding it out into the lumen and worsening stenosis.

Unstable angina may be complicated by impaired coronary vasodilatation, and vasospasm due to plaque-associated endothelial damage, which reduces the local release of endothelium-dependent relaxing factors. Platelet aggregation and thrombosis also cause the local generation of vasoconstrictors such as thromboxane A_2 and serotonin.

Unstable angina as an acute coronary syndrome

Listed in ascending order of severity, unstable angina, non-Q-wave MI and Q-wave MI (Chapter 40) represent the spectrum of **acute coronary syndromes**, i.e. life-threatening events caused by coronary heart disease and resulting in myocardial ischaemia. The pathophysiology of unstable angina is similar to that of acute MI, but less severe. In contrast to patients with acute Q-wave MI, patients with unstable angina do not have complete coronary artery occlusion. Myocardial ischaemia in unstable angina is therefore insufficient to cause **infarction** (tissue death). On coronary angioscopy (visualization of the coronary lumen using a fibreoptic catheter imaging system), the thrombus of unstable angina is usually greyish-white, showing that it is more platelet rich than the red-coloured thrombus of MI.

Diagnosis and prognosis

Transient S–T segment changes or T wave inversion frequently occur on ECG. These are most likely to be seen if the ECG is continuously monitored. Serum levels of C-reactive protein and amyloid-A protein, both markers of inflammation, may be increased. Once symptoms have been controlled by therapy, patients can be given an exercise stress test (see Chapter 37) which indicates their risk of mortality or suffering further acute coronary events. Increased risk is also predicted by the presence of pulmonary oedema, hypotension, mitral regurgitation, diffuse ST depression or left bundle branch block on the ECG, and elevations in serum troponin-T, a marker of myocardial damage.

Within a year of presenting initially with unstable angina, the majority of patients will have adverse events, including another acute coronary syndrome or angiographic total occlusion of the artery, and approximately 10% will die. Those with postinfarction angina represent the highest risk group for 6-month mortality (11%) and re-infarction (20%).

Management

Unstable angina is a medical emergency. Typically, treatment begins with aggressive pharmacological therapy (see Chapter 39) in order to control the symptoms and prevent further acute events. **Urgent revascularization** is considered for patients with high-risk and/or very significant coronary artery disease.

Revascularization

Percutaneous transcoronary angioplasty (PTCA) and **coronary artery bypass grafting** (CABG) are revascularization techniques that are used to treat both stable and unstable angina when symptoms are refractory to medical (pharmacological) therapy. PTCA is a much less invasive procedure, and is preferred when one or two arteries are diseased, and when lesions are amenable to this approach. CABG is used when all three main coronary arteries are diseased (triple-vessel disease), when the left coronary mainstem has a significant stenosis, when the lesion is not amenable to PTCA and when left ventricular function is poor.

CABG is a surgical procedure (Fig. 38.1, lower right). Lengths of healthy superfluous blood vessels (**conduits**) are attached between the aorta and the coronary arteries distal to any stenosis. This allows a supply of blood to the heart, which bypasses the stenosis. Conduits commonly used for CABG include **saphenous vein** segments harvested from the leg. These, however, have limited long-term patency due to early postoperative thrombosis, intimal hyperplasia with smooth muscle proliferation in the first year, and the development of atherosclerosis after approximately 5–7 years. For this reason, the use of arterial grafts such as the **left internal mammary artery** (LIMA) has recently gained popularity. In this case, the LIMA is not disconnected from its parent (subclavian) artery, but is cut distally and attached to the coronary artery. Patients with the LIMA graft to the left anterior descending artery have improved long-term survival compared to patients receiving saphenous vein grafts. The right internal mammary artery, gastro-epiploic artery and radial arteries can also be used for grafting.

In **PTCA**, a guide wire is placed down the lumen of the coronary artery. A balloon catheter is advanced over this wire, and then inflated at the site of the stenosis to increase the lumenal diameter (Fig. 38.1, lower centre). Emergency repeat CABG is required in 1–2% of patients due to acute vessel closure after this procedure. **Restenosis** at the site of the PTCA occurs within 6 months of the procedure in 30% of patients, caused by immediate elastic recoil of the vessel and intimal hyperplasia. The recent use of **stents** has substantially improved acute success and reduced the restenosis rates. Stents are cylindrical metal mesh tubes that are implanted into the artery at the site of balloon expansion following angioplasty. The effect of coronary stenting on long-term survival is as yet unknown.

Benefits of revascularization

Compared with medical therapy, CABG improves survival in patients with severe atherosclerotic disease in all three major coronary arteries or a more than 50% stenosis of the left main coronary artery, particularly if left ventricular function is impaired. Compared to medical therapy, PTCA does not improve survival. However, PTCA results in greater improvement of angina symptoms and exercise tolerance and also diminishes the need for drug therapy. Revascularization must be repeated more often after PTCA compared to CABG.

39 Pharmacological management of angina

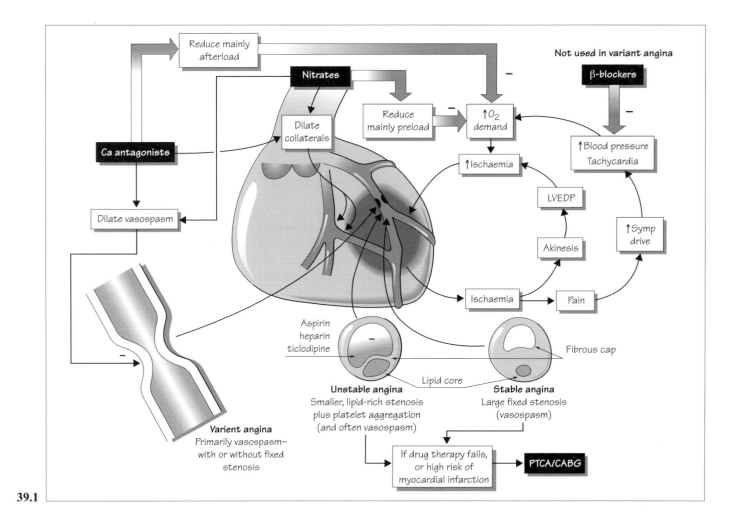

39.1

Angina symptoms are controlled by restoring the balance between myocardial O_2 demand and supply. In **stable angina**, the bloodflow through stenotic coronary arteries is limited, and therapy is mainly aimed at reducing O_2 demand with **vasodilators** and **β-blockers**. These drugs are also used in **unstable angina**, with the addition of aspirin and heparin to inhibit platelet aggregation and thrombosis. The treatment of **variant angina** is primarily directed at reversing coronary **vasospasm**.

Nitrovasodilators

Nitrovasodilators include **nitroglycerin** (glyceryl trinitrate), **isosorbide mononitrate**, **isosorbide dinitrate**, **erythrityl tetranitrate**, and **pentaerythritol tetranitrate**. Nitrovasodilators are used to terminate ongoing angina attacks, and when combined with other drugs also provide prophylaxis.

Nitrovasodilators act as a 'pharmacological endothelium'. They react with cellular thiols (–SH groups) in vascular smooth muscle cells, thereby releasing nitrite ions (NO_2^-). These are then reduced to nitric oxide, which stimulates guanylate cyclase to elevate cGMP, thereby causing vasodilatation (see Chapter 23). At therapeutic doses, nitrovasodilators act primarily to dilate veins, thus reducing central venous pressure (preload), and ventricular end-diastolic volume. This lowers myocardial contraction, wall stress, and O_2 demand. Some arterial dilatation also occurs, diminishing total peripheral resistance (afterload). This allows the left ventricle to maintain cardiac output with a smaller stroke volume, again decreasing O_2 demand.

Nitrovasodilators can also increase the perfusion of ischaemic myocardium by several mechanisms. They dilate coronary **collateral vessels** (see Chapter 3). These often increase in number in the presence of a significant stenosis, providing alternative perfusion of ischaemic zones. Nitrovasodilators also relieve coronary vasospasm, and help to diminish plaque-related platelet aggregation and thrombosis by elevating platelet cGMP.

Nitroglycerin and isosorbide dinitrate taken sublingually relieve angina within minutes; this route of administration avoids extensive first-pass metabolism of these drugs associated with oral dosing. These and other nitrovasodilators can also be given in slowly absorbed oral, transdermal and buccal forms for sustained effect. Continuous exposure to nitrovasodilators causes **tolerance**, which may in part be caused by the depletion of tissue thiols. Tolerance is of no consequence with short-acting nitrovasodilators. With long-acting preparations, tolerance can be minimized by dosing schedules that allow blood concentrations to become low overnight. The most important adverse effect of nitrovasodilators is headache. Reflex tachycardia and orthostatic hypotension may also occur.

Ca²⁺-channel blockers (Ca²⁺ antagonists)

These drugs act by blocking the voltage-gated Ca^{2+} channels that allow depolarization-mediated influx of Ca^{2+} into smooth muscle cells, and also cardiac myocytes (see Chapters 11, 12). The interaction of blocker and Ca^{2+} channel is best understood for the *dihydropyridines*, which include **nifedipine**, **amlodipine**, and **felodipine**. The affinity of dihydropyridines for the channel increases enormously when the channel is in its *inactivated* state (see Chapter 10). Channel inactivation is favoured by a less negative membrane potential (Em). Dihydropyridines therefore have a relatively selective effect on vascular muscle (Em ~–50) compared to cardiac muscle (Em ~–80). This selectivity is further enhanced because dihydropyridine-mediated vasodilatation stimulates the baroreceptor reflex, overcoming direct negative inotropic effects.

The phenylalkylamine **verapamil** interacts preferentially with the channel in its *open* state. Verapamil binding is therefore less dependent on membrane potential; and both cardiac and vascular Ca^{2+} channels are blocked. Verapamil therefore has negative inotropic effects and severely depresses AV nodal conduction. The benzothiazepine **diltiazem** has intermediate properties; at therapeutic doses it vasodilates but also depresses AV conduction and has negative inotropic/chronotropic effects.

The Ca^{2+}-channel blockers prevent angina mainly by causing arteriolar vasodilatation and decreasing afterload. They can also prevent coronary vasospasm, making them particularly useful in variant angina. The negative inotropic and chronotropic effects of verapamil and diltiazem also contribute to their usefulness by reducing myocardial O_2 demand.

The vasodilatation caused by Ca^{2+}-channel blockers can cause hypotension, headache, and peripheral oedema (mainly dihydropyridines). On the other hand, their cardiac effects can elicit excessive cardiodepression and AV node conduction block (mainly verapamil and diltiazem). These drugs are contraindicated in heart failure, especially if β-blockers are being used.

β-Adrenergic receptor blockers

As the figure illustrates, myocardial ischaemia creates a vicious cycle by activating the sympathetic system and increasing ventricular end-diastolic pressure; both these effects then worsen ischaemia and anginal pain. **β-blockers**, which are used for the prophylaxis of angina, help to block this cycle, thereby decreas-

ing O_2 demand. They further reduce O_2 demand by decreasing myocardial contractility and wall stress. The resting and exercising heart rate also falls. This increases the fraction of time the heart spends in diastole, thus enhancing perfusion of the left ventricle, which occurs predominantly during diastole. The properties of β-blockers are further described in Chapter 35.

Drug combinations

Therapy is typically instituted with a short-acting nitrovasodilator taken to terminate attacks. If control is insufficient, a Ca^{2+} antagonist or β-blocker is added for prophylaxis. If necessary, this can be supplemented with a long-acting nitrovasodilator. Finally, a combination of all of these agents can be employed. β-blockers should be given to all unstable angina patients unless contraindicated, since they reduce the risk of myocardial infarction. β-blockers should not be used in variant angina because they may worsen coronary vasospasm.

Aspirin

As described in Chapters 38 and 40, platelet aggregation and thrombosis are critical events in the development of acute coronary syndromes. Clinical trials have confirmed that long-term treatment with **aspirin**, which suppresses platelet aggregation, greatly reduces the risk of myocardial infarction and death in patients with both stable and unstable angina.

Aspirin blocks **cyclooxygenase**, the first enzyme in the branching reaction sequence leading to the formation of the **prostanoids**, including **thromboxane A₂** (TXA_2) and **prostacyclin**. TXA_2 is produced by platelets and promotes platelet aggregation. Prostacyclin is produced by endothelial cells and inhibits platelet aggregation.

Although aspirin directly blocks the formation of both prostanoids, its effect on TXA_2 predominates. This selectivity arises because aspirin inhibits cyclooxygenase *irreversibly*. Following aspirin dosing, levels of both prostacyclin and thromboxane fall, recovering only when new cyclooxygenase is produced via gene transcription and translation. This is impossible in platelets, which lack nuclei (see Chapter 5). TXA_2 production therefore remains depressed for several days, until new platelets are formed. Conversely, endothelial cells can make new cyclooxygenase within hours, allowing rapid recovery of prostacyclin production. Because of this difference in recovery rates, aspirin therapy produces a sustained increase in the prostacyclin/TXA_2 ratio, thereby inhibiting platelet aggregation. Clinical trials have also shown that treatment of unstable angina with intravenous **heparin** reduces the short-term risk of myocardial infarction. The combination of heparin and aspirin is superior to either drug alone, and also helps prevent hypercoagulability and rebound angina, which develop when heparin is withdrawn. **Ticlopidine**, which is thought to block activation of platelets by ADP, can be used in patients with adverse reactions to aspirin. This drug is also particularly useful for preventing the formation of thrombi on newly implanted coronary stents (Chapter 38).

40 Pathophysiology of acute myocardial infarction

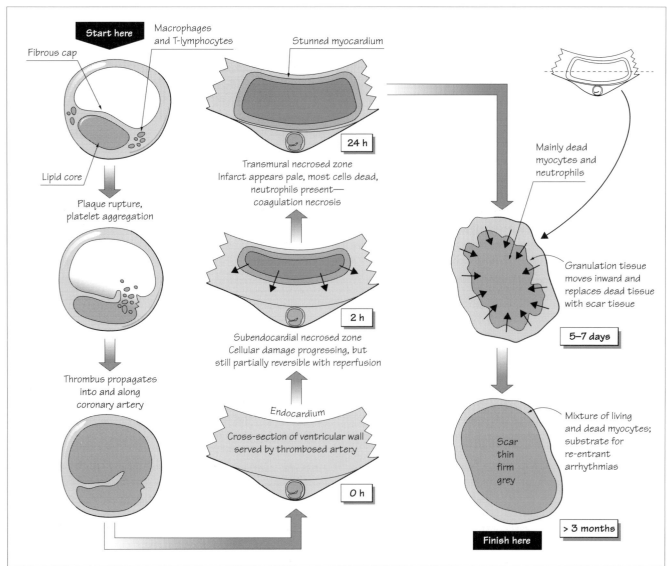

Start here

Fibrous cap

Macrophages and T-lymphocytes

Stunned myocardium

Lipid core

Plaque rupture, platelet aggregation

Transmural necrosed zone
Infarct appears pale, most cells dead, neutrophils present—coagulation necrosis

24 h

Mainly dead myocytes and neutrophils

Thrombus propagates into and along coronary artery

Subendocardial necrosed zone
Cellular damage progressing, but still partially reversible with reperfusion

2 h

Granulation tissue moves inward and replaces dead tissue with scar tissue

5–7 days

Endocardium

Cross-section of ventricular wall served by thrombosed artery

0 h

Scar thin firm grey

Mixture of living and dead myocytes; substrate for re-entrant arrhythmias

> 3 months

Finish here

40.1

Infarction is tissue death caused by ischaemia. Acute **myo-cardial infarction** (MI) occurs when localized myocardial ischaemia causes the development of a defined region of **necrosis** (cell death, with subsequent inflammation and scarring). MI is most often caused by rupture of an atherosclerotic lesion in a coronary artery. This causes the formation of a thrombus that plugs the artery, stopping it from supplying blood to the region of the heart that it supplies.

Role of thrombosis in MI

Pivotal studies by DeWood and colleagues showed that *coronary thrombosis* is the critical event resulting in MI. Of patients presenting within 4 h of symptom onset with ECG evidence

of transmural MI, coronary angiography showed that 87% had complete thrombotic occlusion of the infarct-related artery. The incidence of total occlusion fell to 65% 12–24 h after symptom onset due to spontaneous fibrinolysis. Fresh thrombus on top of ruptured plaque has also been demonstrated in the infarct-related artery in patients dying of MI.

Mechanisms and consequences of plaque rupture

Coronary plaques which are prone to rupture are typically small and nonobstructive, with a large lipid-rich core covered by a thin fibrous cap. Activated **macrophages** and **T lymphocytes** localized at the site of plaque rupture are thought to release **metalloproteases** and **cytokines** which weaken the fibrous cap, rendering it liable to tear or erode due to the shear stress exerted by the bloodflow.

Plaque rupture reveals subendothelial collagen, which serves as a site of platelet adhesion, activation, and aggregation. This results in:

1 The release of substances such as *thromboxane A_2 (TXA$_2$)*, *fibrinogen*, *5-hydroxytryptamine (5-HT)*, *platelet activating factor* and *ADP*, which further promote platelet aggregation.

2 Activation of the clotting cascade, leading to fibrin formation and propagation and stabilization of the occlusive thrombus.

The endothelium is often damaged around areas of coronary artery disease. The resulting deficit of antithrombotic factors such as *thrombomodulin* and *prostacyclin* enhances thrombus formation. In addition, the tendency of several platelet-derived factors (e.g. TXA$_2$, 5-HT) to cause vasoconstriction is increased in the absence of endothelial-derived relaxing factors. This may promote the development of local vasospasm, which worsens coronary occlusion.

Sudden death and acute coronary syndrome onset show a **circadian variation** (daily cycle), peaking at around 9 a.m. with a trough at around 11 p.m. Levels of catecholamines peak about an hour after awakening in the morning, resulting in maximal levels of platelet aggregability, vascular tone, heart rate, and blood pressure, which may trigger plaque rupture and thrombosis. Increased physical and mental stress can also cause MI and sudden death, supporting a role for increases in catecholamines in MI pathophysiology. Furthermore, chronic β-adrenergic receptor blockade abolishes the circadian rhythm of MI.

Autopsies of young subjects killed in road accidents often show small plaque ruptures in susceptible arteries, suggesting that plaque rupture does not always have pathological consequences. The degree of coronary occlusion and myocardial damage caused by plaque rupture probably depends on systemic catecholamine levels, as well as local factors such as plaque location and morphology, the depth of plaque rupture, and the extent to which coronary vasoconstriction occurs. Infarct size depends on factors such as the extent and duration of occlusion, the site of occlusion within the coronary arterial tree, the degree to which a collateral circulation exists, and also the level of oxygen demand in the affected zone of myocardium.

Severe and prolonged ischaemia produces a region of necrosis spanning the entire thickness of the myocardial wall. Such a *transmural* infarct often causes S–T segment elevation, and the development of an exaggerated Q wave on the ECG, in which case it is termed a **Q wave MI** (see Fig. 40.1). Less severe and protracted ischaemia can arise when:

1 Coronary occlusion is followed by spontaneous reperfusion.

2 The infarct-related artery is not completely occluded.

3 Occlusion is complete, but an existing collateral blood supply prevents complete ischaemia. This results in a necrotic zone which is mainly limited to the subendocardium, typically causing a **non-Q wave (nontransmural) MI**, after which the Q wave remains unaltered, and S–T segment depression often occurs.

Evolution of the infarct

Both infarcted and unaffected myocardial regions undergo progressive changes over the hours, days and weeks following coronary thrombosis. This process of postinfarct myocardial evolution leads to the occurrence of characteristic complications at predictable times after the initial event (see Chapter 41).

Ischaemia causes an immediate loss of contractility in the affected myocardium. Necrosis starts to develop in the subendocardium (which is most prone to ischaemia; see Chapter 37), about 15–30 min after coronary occlusion. The necrotic region grows outward towards the epicardium over the next 3–6 h, eventually spanning the entire ventricular wall. In some areas (generally at the edges of the infarct) the myocardium is **stunned** (reversibly damaged) and will eventually recover if bloodflow is restored. Contractility in the remaining viable myocardium increases, a process termed **hyperkinesis**.

A progression of cellular, histological and gross changes develop within the infarct. Although alterations in the gross appearance of infarcted tissue are not apparent for at least 6 h after the onset of cell death, cell biochemistry and ultrastructure begin to show abnormalities within 20 min. Cell damage is progressive, becomingly increasingly irreversible over about 12 h. This period therefore provides a window of opportunity, during which thrombolysis and reperfusion may salvage some of the infarct (see Chapter 41).

Between 4 and 12 h after cell death starts, the infarcted myocardium begins to undergo **coagulation necrosis**, a process characterized by cell swelling, organelle breakdown, and protein denaturation. After about 18 h, **neutrophils** (phagocytic lymphocytes) enter the infarct. Their numbers reach a peak after about 5 days, and then decline. After 3–4 days, **granulation tissue** appears at the edges of the infarct zone. This consists of **macrophages**, **fibroblasts**, which lay down scar tissue, and **new capillaries**. The infarcted myocardium is especially soft between 4 and 7 days, and is therefore maximally prone to **rupturing**. This event is usually fatal, may occur at any time during the first 2 weeks and is responsible for about 10% of MI mortality. As the granulation tissue migrates inward toward the centre of the infarct over several weeks, the necrotic tissue is engulfed and digested by the macrophages. The granulation tissue then progressively matures, with an increase in connective (scar) tissue and loss of capillaries. After 2–3 months, the infarct has healed, leaving a noncontracting region of the ventricular wall that is thinned, firm, and pale grey.

Infarct expansion, the stretching and thinning of the infarcted wall, may occur within the first day or so after a MI. Over the course of several months, there is progressive dilatation, not only of the infarct zone, but also of healthy myocardium. This process of **ventricular remodelling** is caused by an increase in end-diastolic wall stress. Infarct expansion puts patients at a substantial risk for the development of congestive heart failure, ventricular arrhythmias, and free wall rupture. Factors promoting infarct expansion include transmural infarction, anterior location, 100% occlusion of the infarct vessel, and a large infarction.

41 Clinical aspects of acute myocardial infarction

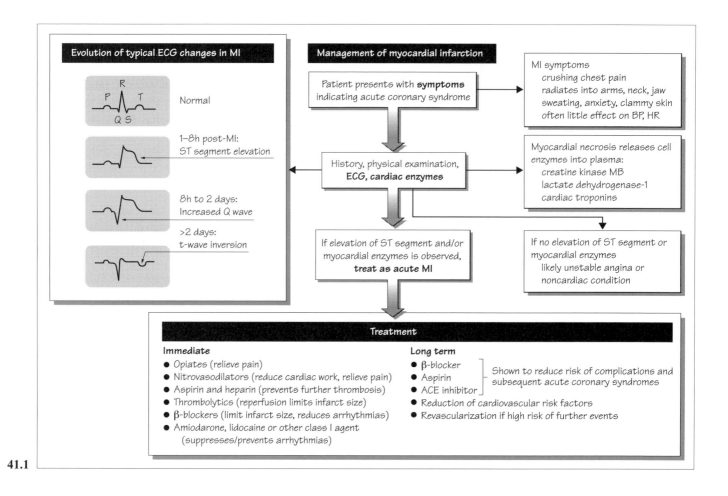

41.1

Symptoms and signs

Patients present with central crushing chest pain, which may radiate into the arms, jaw, or neck. The pain lasts > 30 min and is not relieved by nitroglycerin. The patient is frequently sweating and may appear cold and clammy. Nausea or vomiting and intense feelings of anxiety are common. Some individuals present atypically, with no symptoms (**silent infarction**, most common in diabetic subjects), unusual locations of the pain, syncope, or peripheral embolization. The pulse may demonstrate a tachycardia or bradycardia. The blood pressure is usually normal. However, a systolic pressure of < 90 mmHg, and evidence of organ hypoperfusion herald **cardiogenic shock** (see Chapter 30). The rest of the examination of the cardiovascular system may be remarkably normal, but there may be a third or fourth sound audible on ascultation as well as systolic murmur.

Complications

With large infarctions (> 20–25% of the left ventricle (LV)), depression of pump function is sufficient to cause **cardiac failure**. An infarction involving > 40% of the LV causes car-diogenic shock. **Rupture** of the free LV wall (see Chapter 40) is almost always fatal. Rupture of the ventricular septum may result in leakage of blood between the ventricles. Rupture of the myocardium underlying a papillary muscle, or more rarely of the papillary muscle itself, may cause **mitral regurgitation**. **Arrhythmias** in the acute phase include ventricular ectopic beats, ventricular tachycardia, or ventricular fibrillation. Supraventricular arrhythmias include atrial ectopics, flutter, and fibrillation. Bradyarrhythmias are also common, including sinus bradycardia, and first-, second- and third-degree AV block. **Infarct expansion** (see Chapter 40) is a dangerous late complication.

Investigations

ECG changes associated with MI indicate the site, extent and thickness (Q-wave or non-Q-wave) of the infarct. S–T segment abnormalities, increased Q-waves and inversion of the T-wave typically evolve in transmural MI as shown in Fig. 41.1. A more than twofold elevation of plasma concentrations of certain cardiac cellular enzymes indicates that myocardial necrosis has occurred. These include **creatine kinase-MB** (CK-MB), **lactate** dehydrogenase-1 (LDH_1), and **cardiac troponins T** and **I**. CK-MB levels begin to rise within 4–8 h, peak at 24 h, and decline to normal at 2–3 days. LDH_1 levels begin to rise at 24–48 h, peak at 3–6 days, and return to normal at 8–14 days. The cardiac troponins begin to rise within 4–8 h and remain elevated for 4–7 days.

Management
Immediate management
Patients with suspected MI should be assessed using a 12-lead ECG, and by brief history and examination, and should be put on bed-rest and oxygen. All patients with suspected MI should receive **aspirin** to block further platelet aggregation. **Opiates** are generally used to relieve pain. **Nitrovasodilators** may also help to reduce cardiac work and control pain. **β-blockers** should be used unless there are contraindications. Patients with S–T elevation of more than 1 mm in two contiguous leads (indicates Q-wave MI), or new left bundle branch block, should undergo **thrombolysis**.

Subseqent management
Long-term treatment with aspirin, β-blockers and **ACE inhibitors** reduces both the complications of MI and the risk of re-infarction. Cessation of smoking, treatment of hypertension and diabetes, and reduction of lipids using HMG-CoA reductase inhibitors (Chapter 33) are vital. Individuals with continuing angina following MI are at high risk of further events and should undergo early revascularization. Patients should undergo exercise stress testing prior to hospital discharge. If this indicates that the risk of further events is high, these individuals should be referred for angiography and revascularization.

Thrombolytic agents
Thrombolysis is the dissolution of the blood clot plugging the infarct-related coronary artery. This leads to reperfusion of the infarct zone. Reperfusion limits infarct size and reduces the risk of complications such as infarct expansion, arrhythmias and cardiac failure. Clinical trials have demonstrated that thrombolytic agents reduce mortality by about 25% in MI when the ECG shows S–T elevation or left bundle branch block. However, patients without S–T elevation (indicates non-Q-wave MI) do not benefit from thrombolysis. It is critical that thrombolysis is instituted as quickly as possible. Although significant reductions in short-term mortality occur when thrombolytics are given within 12 h of symptom onset, the greatest benefits occur when therapy is instituted within 3 h. The main risk of thrombolysis is bleeding, particularly intracerebral haemorrhage (stroke). Contraindications to thrombolytic therapy include prior stroke, active ulcers, and recent surgery.

Thrombolytic (fibrinolytic) agents act by inducing **fibrinolysis**, the lysis (fragmentation) of the fibrin strands holding the clot together. Fibrinolysis normally occurs when the inactive proenzyme **plasminogen** is converted to the active fibrinolytic enzyme **plasmin** by the endogenous endothelium-derived **tissue plasminogen activator (t-PA)**. Plasmin also inactivates fibrinogen, and coagulation factors V and VIII.

Streptokinase (SK) is a bacterial protein that is inactive until it binds a molecule of plasminogen. This complex then cleaves other plasminogen molecules to produce plasmin. SK has a plasma clearance time of 15–25 min. It activates plasminogen both in the plasma, and on clots, so it can cause haemorrhage. Streptokinase can only be used once since it may produce antibodies that can cause significant allergic reactions. **t-PA** (alteplase) is produced commercially by recombinant DNA technology. t-PA binds to fibrin, so it has a greater effect on clot-associated plasminogen than on plasma plasminogen. t-PA is cleared from the plasma within 4–8 min, and is not antigenic. **u-PA** (urokinase) is another endogenous plasminogen activator with properties similar to those of t-PA. **Anistreplase (APSAC)** is a complex of human plasminogen and SK which is rendered inactive by the addition of an anisoyl group to the streptokinase. This group is removed slowly in plasma, freeing SK to activate plasminogen. Similar to SK, APSAC is antigenic and may cause allergic reactions. APSAC has a long plasma clearance time of 50–90 min.

Other drugs used in myocardial infarct
Antiplatelet and **anticoagulant** therapy is used after MI to prevent further platelet aggregation and thrombosis in the infarct-related artery. **Aspirin** inhibits platelet aggregation (see Chapter 39). The 2nd International Trial of Infarct Survival (ISIS-II) demonstrated a 23% reduction in 35-day mortality in patients randomized to 160 mg/day of aspirin. Aspirin combined with SK had a *synergistic benefit* compared to placebo (42% reduction). 160–325 mg of aspirin should be given daily to all patients to prevent vessel occlusion and infarction. Because t-PA is more fibrin specific and has a shorter half-life than SK, intravenous heparin for a duration of 48–72 h should be used when this agent is administered. Unless contraindicated, subcutaneous low-dose heparin should be used in all infarct patients to prevent deep vein thrombosis and pulmonary emboli.

β-blockers are beneficial in MI for several reasons. They diminish oxygen demand by lowering heart rate and decrease ventricular wall stress by lowering afterload. β-blockers therefore reduce ischaemia and infarct size when given acutely. They also decrease recurrent ischaemia, free wall rupture and suppress arrhythmias (Chapters 39, 46). Long-term oral β-blockade reduces mortality, recurrent MI and sudden death by about 25%.

ACE inhibitors reduce afterload and ventricular wall stress and improve ejection fraction. Inhibition of ACE raises bradykinin levels, which may improve endothelial function and limit coronary vasospasm. ACE inhibitors also limit ventricular remodelling and infarct expansion (Chapter 40), thereby reducing mortality and the incidence of congestive heart failure and recurrent MI. Therapy should be instituted immediately in patients with Q-wave MI or evidence of heart failure, and should continue long term if evidence of LV dysfunction is present.

42 Emerging approaches to therapy of coronary artery disease

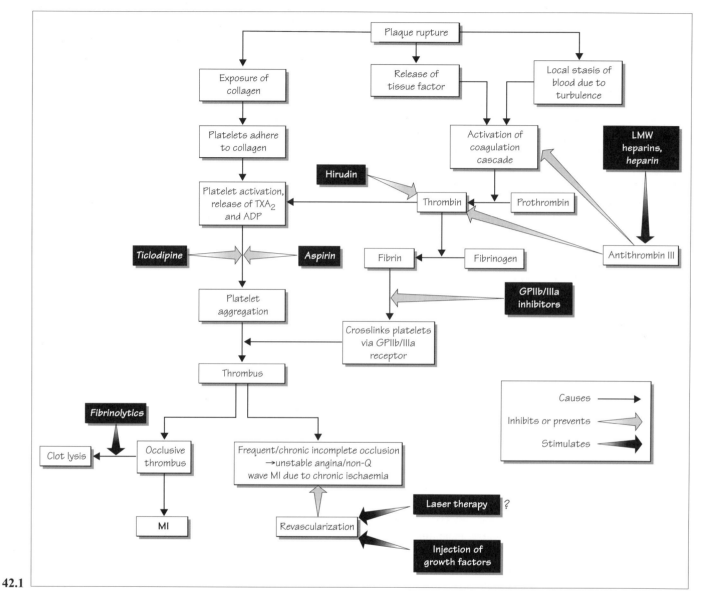

42.1

Acute coronary syndromes such as unstable angina and non-Q-wave MI are typically caused by plaque rupture, with activation of platelets and thrombosis (see Chapters 38, 40). Aspirin therapy has been demonstrated to reduce the risk of recurrent MI and death in patients with acute coronary syndromes. Aspirin, however, is a relatively weak inhibitor of platelet aggregation. Although it blocks cyclooxygenase-dependent platelet aggregation, it does not inhibit platelet aggregation to other mediators, such as ADP, collagen, and low thrombin concentrations. Unlike aspirin and also heparin, conventional thrombolytics appear to be of little value in unstable angina. For example, the Thrombolysis in Myocardial Infarction (TIMI) IIIb Study found

that adding thrombolytic therapy to aspirin and heparin did not decrease short-term mortality, and increased the risk of suffering MI in patients with unstable angina. The increased risk may have been from the platelet activation that occurs with such therapy. Newer agents targeting other antithrombotic mechanisms are therefore currently being evaluated.

Glycoprotein IIb/IIIa inhibitors

The final common pathway to platelet aggregation is the binding of fibrinogen to the activated platelet receptor **glycoprotein (GP) IIb/IIIa**. This receptor is the most abundant on platelets and, when activated, avidly binds fibrinogen and von

Willebrand's factor, which form crosslinks between platelets, leading to aggregation. Powerful platelet inhibitors have been developed which either competitively inhibit the GPIIb/IIIa receptor or, as a monoclonal antibody, bind to the receptor and prevent platelet aggregation.

Recent clinical trials have evaluated GPIIb/IIIa antagonists, which include **tirofiban**, **eptifibatide**, and **abciximab**. In patients undergoing high-risk angioplasty, such as in the setting of unstable angina or recent MI, the addition of GPIIb/IIIa blockade to aspirin and heparin significantly reduces the short-term risk of death, MI, and the need for urgent revascularization due to refractory symptoms. These agents are well tolerated with no significant increased risk of major bleeding compared to placebo-treated patients. One of the limitations of this current therapy is its availability only as an intravenous infusion. Ongoing trials in patients with acute coronary syndromes are evaluating oral GPIIb/IIIa inhibitors for longer duration of treatment.

New approaches to inhibiting thrombin: can heparin be improved upon?

Patients with acute coronary syndromes often demonstrate hypercoagulability (see Chapter 7). Anticoagulation therapy with intravenous heparin has been demonstrated to reduce MI and refractory angina in patients with unstable angina. Conventional unfractionated heparin is a mixture of mucopolysaccharides with molecular weights between 3 and 40 kDa. It prevents coagulation by activating antithrombin III, a naturally occurring plasma protein that inactivates thrombin and clotting factors Xa, IXa, XIa, and XIIa. Heparin, however, has several drawbacks as an anticoagulant. Firstly, it does not affect the activity of thrombin or factor Xa which are clot bound. Secondly, studies in patients with unstable angina show that following discontinuation of heparin, there is a rebound in clinical events, such as MI and refractory angina. This is likely to be due to a rebound in hypercoagulability. Thirdly, unfractionated heparin is inactivated by platelet factor 4 and has variable protein binding, resulting in large intra- and interpatient variability of heparin dosing. Finally, between 5 and 15% of patients on heparin develop **thrombocytopenia** (reduced platelet numbers).

Low-molecular-weight heparins (LMWH) include **enoxaparin**, **dalteparin**, **nadroparin**, **reviparin**, **tinzaparin**, and **ardeparin**. LMWH are one-third the molecular weight of standard unfractionated heparin, and have several advantages over their parent molecule. These substances are minimally bound to plasma proteins, are not inactivated by platelet factor 4, and have a longer plasma half-life. These properties result in a predictable dose–response relationship. LMWH inhibit factor Xa to a greater degree than thrombin. This has the benefit of allowing anticoagulation without a prolongation of the activated partial-thromboplastin time (APTT). The APTT is an indication of the degree of anticoagulation, and is increased by heparin. Because heparin preparations are heterogeneous, the dose of heparin must be adjusted for each patient by measuring the APPT. This is not necessary with LMWH. These drugs are injected subcutaneously and are potentially suitable for outpatient use. Finally, LMWH cause less risk of thrombocytopenia compared to heparin.

The Efficacy and Safety of Subcutaneous Enoxaparin in Non-Q-Wave Coronary Events Trail compared enoxaparin to unfractionated heparin in patients admitted to hospital with unstable angina or non-Q-wave MI. All patients received aspirin. The combined primary endpoints of death, MI or recurrent angina at 14 days were significantly reduced by 16% in the patients randomized to enoxaparin. Trials are ongoing to determine if longer-term use of LMWH is well tolerated and has further benefits.

Hirudin is a 65-amino-acid protein originally discovered in the medicinal leech *Hirudo medicinalis*, and now synthesized by recombinant DNA techniques. Unlike heparin, hirudin inhibits thrombin directly. It can act on clot-bound thrombin, and results in consistent anticoagulation. The Global Use of Strategies to Open Occluded Arteries (GUSTO) IIb Trial compared 72 h of treatment with heparin or hirudin in patients presenting to hospital within 12 h of chest pain and acute coronary syndromes. All patients also received aspirin. The primary endpoint of this study, death within 30 days or nonfatal MI, occurred in 9.8% of heparin-treated patients and 8.9% of hirudin-treated patients. This result was of borderline statistical significance, and has prompted a further similar trial which is currently in progress.

New approaches to revascularization

Transmyocardial laser revascularization involves using a laser to drill 20–40 small channels through the wall of the ischaemic myocardium. The channels heal at their epicardial ends, otherwise remaining open. This experimental technique has been used in patients with refractory angina who are not candidates for conventional revascularization, and appears to relieve symptoms in most cases. The mechanism by which it does so remains unknown, but it might involve stimulation of new blood vessel growth (angiogenesis). **Angiogenic gene therapy** is a novel approach to producing angiogenesis. Investigators have treated patients with critical lower extremity ischaemia (ischaemia of the legs producing rest pain and/or ulceration) with intramuscular injection of bacterial plasmid DNA into which the gene for human **vascular endothelial growth factor** is inserted. This **mitogen** (growth stimulator) for vascular endothelial cells resulted in improved lower extremity perfusion in these patients. In a recent report, investigators induced neoangiogenesis by injecting **human basic fibroblast growth factor** into areas of ischaemic myocardium of patients during coronary artery bypass surgery. Follow-up angiograms demonstrated new vessel growth around the site of injection. This exciting work of inducing angiogenesis in areas of ischaemic myocardium has resulted in several ongoing trials in patients with severe coronary artery disease.

43 Chronic heart failure

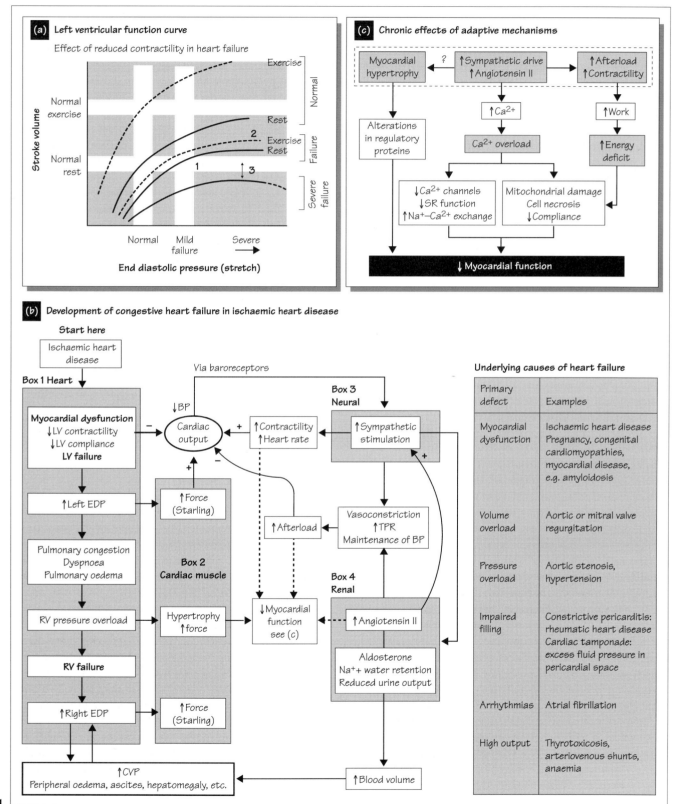

(a) Left ventricular function curve

Effect of reduced contractility in heart failure

(c) Chronic effects of adaptive mechanisms

(b) Development of congestive heart failure in ischaemic heart disease

Underlying causes of heart failure

Primary defect	Examples
Myocardial dysfunction	Ischaemic heart disease Pregnancy, congenital cardiomyopathies, myocardial disease, e.g. amyloidosis
Volume overload	Aortic or mitral valve regurgitation
Pressure overload	Aortic stenosis, hypertension
Impaired filling	Constrictive pericarditis; rheumatic heart disease Cardiac tamponade: excess fluid pressure in pericardial space
Arrhythmias	Atrial fibrillation
High output	Thyrotoxicosis, arteriovenous shunts, anaemia

43.1

In **heart failure**, the heart is unable to produce an adequate cardiac output to perfuse the tissues, or can do so only with an elevated filling pressure. Initially adaptive mechanisms may compensate and so maintain cardiac output at rest, although they may not be sufficient to allow normal increases in output during exercise. In spite of these mechanisms cardiac function eventually declines, and heart failure becomes severe (**decompensated heart failure**). Heart failure can be precipitated by other acute diseases or stresses.

Systolic failure is a defect in systolic function that impairs ejection, whereas **diastolic failure** is a defect in ventricular filling. Systolic and diastolic failure often coexist, particularly in **ischaemic heart disease**.

Clinical manifestations of heart failure

Patients generally suffer from **dyspnoea** (breathlessness) though initially only during exercise, weakness, fatigue, and **peripheral oedema** (fluid retention in tissues, see Chapter 20). The heart and liver are enlarged, and a high venous pressure distends the jugular veins. The **ejection fraction** (proportion of EDV ejected per beat) is reduced early in the development of heart failure.

Pathophysiology of chronic heart failure

Many conditions can lead to heart failure (see Fig. 43.1, lower right). The most common cause is dysfunction of cardiac muscle (**myocardium**) due to **ischaemic heart disease**. Coronary bloodflow and oxygen delivery are insufficient for the needs of the myocardium, leading to dysfunction. The force developed for any degree of stretch (**contractility**, see Chapter 14) is reduced, and the ventricular function curve is depressed (Fig. 43.1a). In mild failure, acceptable output can only be obtained at rest with an increased end-diastolic pressure (EDP) (**1**). In exercise the function curve can never reach the required output (**2**); the increase in contractility is small because sympathetic tone is already high (see below). In severe failure normal resting output cannot be obtained even with substantial increases in EDP (**3**).

Left heart failure

Ischaemic heart disease most commonly affects the left ventricle. In left heart failure decreased output leads to an increased left ventricular EDP and pulmonary venous pressure (Fig. 43.1b, Box 1). This results in **pulmonary congestion**, fluid accumulation in the interstitium of the lungs and pleural spaces (**pleural effusion**), and thus **dyspnoea**. Dyspnoea may only occur when the patient lies down (**orthopnoea**) or at night (**paroxysmal dyspnoea**), when redistribution of body fluids allows fluid to collect in the lungs. If severe, fluid enters the alveoli (**pulmonary oedema**), this causes extreme dyspnoea, and can 'drown' the patient by reducing gas exchange. In severe pulmonary oedema the patient is always breathless and hypoxaemic, and very occasionally produces pinkish foam at the lips.

Right heart failure

Right heart failure occurs in chronic lung disease (**cor pulmonale**), pulmonary hypertension or embolism, and valve disease of the right heart. Central venous pressure (CVP) is greatly increased, with consequent **distension of the jugular veins, enlarged heart, peripheral oedema**, fluid accumulation in the peritoneum (**ascites**), and **tenderness and enlargement of the liver** (**hepatomegaly**). Ambulatory patients show **pitting oedema** of the ankles (a depression is left following compression with a finger), which is relieved on lying down.

Congestive heart failure (Fig. 43.1b, Box 1)

Left heart failure can cause subsequent failure of the right heart due to the greatly increased pulmonary vascular pressure. The right ventricle will initially develop **hypertrophy** against the increased afterload, but eventually it fails due to pressure overload. This is known as **congestive heart failure**.

Compensatory mechanisms: 'the good, the bad and the ugly'

Adaptive mechanisms may initially compensate for reduced function, but are commonly deleterious when sustained. All increase cardiac work and thus oxygen requirement, which is clearly detrimental in ischaemic heart disease.

Starling's Law

A decrease in myocardial force or increase in afterload results in a **reduced ejection fraction**. Thus more blood is left in the ventricle at the end of systole, leading to increased EDV. There is a rightward shift along the ventricular function curve, and force increases due to **Starling's Law** (Fig. 43.1a; Fig. 43.1b, Box 2; see Chapter 14).

Cardiac dilatation

A greatly increased EDV causes **cardiac dilatation**. Coupled with reduced function this is described as a **dilated cardiomyopathy**. Dilatation reduces the *efficiency* of the heart from application of the **Law of Laplace**. This states that pressure is proportional to wall tension (i.e. muscle force) divided by the radius of the lumen. Thus grossly dilated hearts have to contract harder in order to develop normal pressures.

Neurohumoral systems

Low blood pressure initiates the **baroreceptor reflex**, and stimulates the sympathetic nervous system (Fig. 43.1b, Box 3; see Chapter 27). This increases heart rate (**tachycardia**) and contractility, and improves cardiac output (see Chapters 11, 14). It also causes vasoconstriction, increasing total peripheral resistance (TPR) and helping to maintain blood pressure. This however, increases afterload, and redistribution of output from skeletal muscle and splanchnic circulations leads to muscle weakness and fatigue, impaired renal function, and in severe cases renal necrosis. These effects may be limited later in the disease because β-adrenoceptor density falls, and sensitivity to norepinephrine decreases.

Vasoconstriction of renal arteries (Fig. 43.1b, Box 4)

This reduces filtration and urine production, and causes the release of **renin**. Renin activates **angiotensin I**, which is converted in the lungs to **angiotensin II**, a powerful vasoconstrictor that also potentiates sympathetic activity. Angiotensin II stimulates the adrenals to produce **aldosterone**, which augments renal reabsorption of Na+. The consequent fluid retention increases blood volume and CVP. **Vasopressin** (antidiuretic hormone) is also increased, leading to further water retention. The increase in CVP underlies many symptoms of heart failure, e.g. **peripheral oedema** and **dyspnoea**.

Myocardial hypertrophy

A sustained increase in ventricular wall stress (tension/wall thickness) causes cardiac muscle cells to grow larger, and muscle mass to increase (**myocardial hypertrophy**). Although hypertrophy increases ventricular force, it also reduces **compliance** (flexibility), which is further reduced by increased collagen content. The ventricle therefore stretches less as EDP is increased, so reducing the effectiveness of Starling's Law. Hypertrophy is associated with a shift in regulatory proteins (***troponin, tropomyosin, myosin light chain***) towards fetal isoforms, which may decrease contraction velocity and contractility (Fig. 43.1c).

Hypertrophy reduces capillary density, with loss of **coronary reserve** (maximum – basal flow) and reduced perfusion in exercise. This is exacerbated by tachycardia, as the diastolic interval, and therefore coronary bloodflow, is reduced. Gross hypertrophy may also cause defective valve operation.

Myocardial dysfunction caused by heart failure

An important component of the transition to full heart failure is a gradual reduction in myocardial function. This is partly related to the energy deficit and Ca^{2+} overload caused by compensatory mechanisms (Fig. 43.1c). Changes in sarcoplasmic reticulum Ca^{2+} handling are probably responsible for reversal of the **Treppe effect** (see Chapter 11) that is sometimes seen in heart failure, when an increased heart rate can *reduce* tension. Ca^{2+} overload may also lead to arrhythmias.

44 Treatment of chronic heart failure

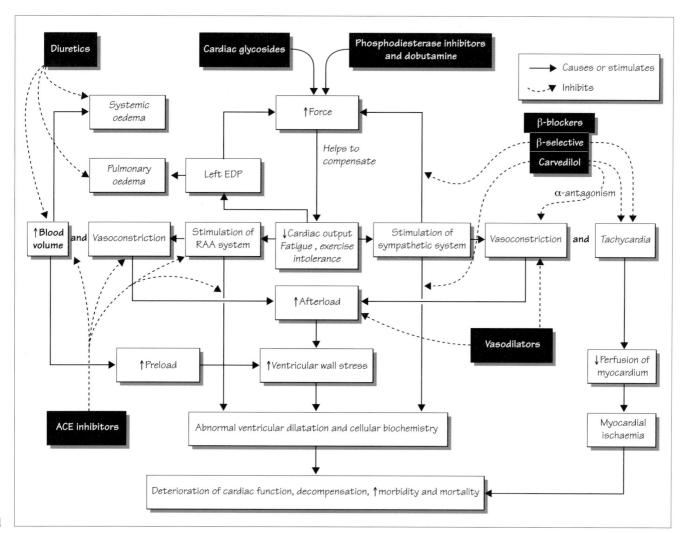

44.1

Therapy of chronic heart failure (CHF) is designed to: (i) improve the quality of life by reducing symptoms; (ii) lengthen survival; and (iii) slow progression of cardiac deterioration. CHF typically has an underlying cause such as ischaemic heart disease, and may be exacerbated by specific **precipitating factors** such as infection or arrhythmias, as well as by myocardial abnormalities which develop as CHF progresses (e.g. valvular dysfunction due to ventricular dilatation). In addition to treating the symptoms of CHF per se, both underlying and precipitating factors should, if possible, be treated. The **sympathetic** and **renin–angiotensin–aldosterone** systems activated in response to reduced pump function initially help to maintain cardiac output (upper part of the figure), but also drive the progression of cardiac deterioration (lower part of the figure; see also Chapter 43). Therapy increasingly involves inhibiting these systems.

Asymptomatic/mild CHF is mainly treated with **angiotensin-converting enzyme inhibitors** (ACEI), which slow CHF progression, lengthen survival time, and improve haemodynamic parameters. *Restricting activity* and *reducing dietary sodium* help to lessen cardiac workload and fluid retention.

In *symptomatic/moderate CHF* a **diuretic** can be given in addition to an ACEI. **Digoxin** is often used to support cardiac function and reduce symptoms. The β-blocker **carvedilol** is increasingly being used to treat mild to moderate CHF.

In *severe or refractory CHF*, or when existing therapy fails to control symptoms adequately, vasodilators such as **hydralazine** and **isosorbide dinitrate** can be added. Positive inotropes such as **dobutamine**, **dopamine** or **milrinone** may be used temporarily if decompensation occurs.

ACEI and other vasodilators

ACEI inhibit conversion of angiotensin I to angiotensin II

(see Chapter 28). Angiotensin II causes *vasoconstriction* by: (i) stimulating the sympathetic nervous system; (ii) increasing norepinephrine release by sympathetic nerves; and (iii) directly constricting vascular smooth muscle. Angiotensin II also *promotes fluid retention* and oedema by directly enhancing renal Na^+ reabsorption, and stimulating aldosterone release. ACEI therefore dilate arteries and veins, and reduce blood volume and oedema. Arterial vasodilatation decreases afterload and cardiac work, and improves tissue perfusion by increasing stroke volume and cardiac output. Venous dilatation and reduction of fluid retention diminish pulmonary congestion, oedema, and central venous pressure (CVP) (preload). Reduction of preload lowers ventricular filling pressure, therefore lowering cardiac wall stress, workload, and ischaemia. ACEI also delay abnormal cardiac hypertrophy and fibrosis, which are thought to be promoted by angiotensin II.

Other vasodilators can be used in patients unable to tolerate the cough or renal dysfunction occasionally caused by ACEI. The ELITE trial reported in 1997 that the angiotensin AT_1 receptor antagonist **losartan** did not cause cough and was as effective as captopril in reducing mortality in elderly heart failure patients. The combination of the nitrovasodilator isosorbide dinitrate (see Chapter 39) and hydralazine is reported to prolong survival, although not as effectively as ACEI. Hydralazine causes mainly arterial vasodilatation, possibly via inhibition of Ca^{2+} release from the sarcoplasmic reticulum. **Nitroprusside** reduces preload and afterload and is given intravenously in acute heart failure.

Cardiac glycosides

Cardiac glycosides include ouabain, digitoxin, and **digoxin**, which is used most widely. Digoxin inhibits the Na^+ pump in cardiac muscle, thereby indirectly inhibiting the Na^+–Ca^{2+} antiport and thus increasing intracellular Ca^{2+} (see Chapter 11). The rise in Ca^{2+}:

1 Enhances contractility.
2 Shortens action potential duration and refractory period in atrial and ventricular cells by stimulating K^+ channels.
3 Often blunts the baroreceptor reflex in CHF, causing sympathetic activation. Digoxin has been shown to increase baroreceptor responsiveness, thereby reducing sympathetic tone.

Digoxin also acts on the nervous system to increase vagal tone. This slows sinoatrial node (SAN) activity and atrioventricular node (AVN) conduction, and can be useful in treating atrial arrhythmias (see Chapter 47).

Digoxin improves CHF symptoms, but does not prolong life. It is mainly used in patients with both CHF and atrial fibrillation.

Digoxin toxicity

Only a two- to threefold excess of digoxin over the optimal therapeutic concentration can cause arrhythmias:

1 An excessive rise in $[Ca^{2+}]_i$ causes oscillations in membrane potential after action potentials. These **delayed afterdepolarizations** can trigger ectopic beats, and at higher doses ventricular tachycardia.

2 Inhibition of the Na^+ pump also decreases intracellular K^+, causing depolarization and facilitating arrhythmias.
3 Excessive vagal tone can block conduction at the AVN.
4 At toxic doses sympathetic tone is increased, again favouring arrhythmias.

Digoxin toxicity is enhanced by **hypokalaemia** (low plasma K^+), because K^+ decreases the affinity of digoxin for the Na^+ pump. Digoxin also causes toxic gastrointestinal effects, including anorexia, nausea, and vomiting. More rarely, visual disturbances, headache and delirium occur. Acute toxicity can be treated with intravenous K^+, antiarrhythmics (e.g. lidocaine), and digoxin-specific antibodies.

Other positive inotropes

Several positive inotropes are used intravenously and for short periods to treat refractory or decompensated heart failure. These drugs are arrhythmogenic and increase myocardial oxygen consumption, and their long-term use is not beneficial. **Dobutamine** acts as a β_1-agonist and α-antagonist, and therefore increases myocardial contractility and decreases afterload. **Dopamine** is also a β_1-agonist, and additionally causes a diuresis by dilating renal arterioles. **Milrinone** and **enoximone** enhance cardiac contractility and vasodilate by blocking phosphodiesterase type III, causing an increase in intracellular cAMP (see Chapters 11, 12).

Diuretics

Diuretics reduce fluid accumulation by increasing renal salt and water excretion. Preload, pulmonary congestion and systemic oedema are thereby relieved. **Loop diuretics** inhibit the $Na^+/K^+/2Cl^-$ symport in the thick ascending loop of Henle. Na^+ and Cl^- reabsorption is thereby inhibited, and the retention of these ions in the tubule promotes fluid loss in the urine. Diuretics are commonly used in CHF, and include **furosemide**, **bumetanide**, **piretanide**, **torasemide**, and **ethacrynic acid**. Thiazide and thiazide-related diuretics (Chapter 35) are also used to treat heart failure.

Both loop and thiazide diuretics can cause hypokalaemia and metabolic alkalosis because the increased Na^+ retained in the tubular fluid is partly exchanged for K^+ and H^+ in the distal nephron. This process is stimulated by aldosterone (see Chapter 28), and diuretic-induced hypokalaemia can be controlled by an ACEI or **spironolactone**, an aldosterone antagonist. Hypokalaemia can also be treated with K^+ supplements, or the use of **K^+-sparing diuretics** such as **amiloride** or **triamterine**. These inhibit Na^+ reabsorption in the collecting duct. Long-term use of loop diuretics can result in hypovolaemia, reduced plasma Mg^{2+}, Ca^{2+} and Na^+, and hyperuricaemia and hyperglycaemia. This is more common in the elderly, who may require high doses of diuretics to overcome **diuretic resistance**.

β-receptor blockers

The 1993 MDC study reported that the β_1-selective antagonist **metoprolol** reduced mortality when added to conventional therapy for mild-to-moderate CHF. The benefits of adding metoprolol to standard therapy (ACE-I and diuretics) were confirmed in the 1999 MERIT-HF study, which showed that this drug reduced 1 year mortality by 34% in patients with mild to severe CHF. **Bisoprolol**, another β_1-selective antagonist, was shown by the 1999 CIBIS-II trial to similarly diminish mortality. **Carvedilol**, a non-selective β-blocker which is also an α-antagonist and anti-oxidant has also been found to prolong survival when added to conventional therapy.

Long-term treatment with β-blockers has been shown to increase ejection fraction, reduce systolic and diastolic volume, and eventually cause regression of left ventricular hypertrophy. Other beneficial effects of β-blockers in CHF probably include reduced ischaemia, a reduction in heart rate so improving myocardial perfusion and inhibition of the deleterious effects of excess catecholamines on myocardial structure and metabolism. β-blockers appear to be particularly effective in reducing sudden death in those with CHF, suggesting that prevention of *ventricular fibrillation* (Chapter 46) constitutes an important part of their action.

The negative inotropic effect of β-blockers is potentially hazardous in some patients with CHF, since cardiac function is already compromised. Therapy is therefore initiated with low doses which are carefully elevated over several weeks or months. Ongoing clinical trials should establish the optimal use of β-blockers in CHF therapy.

45 Mechanisms of arrhythmia

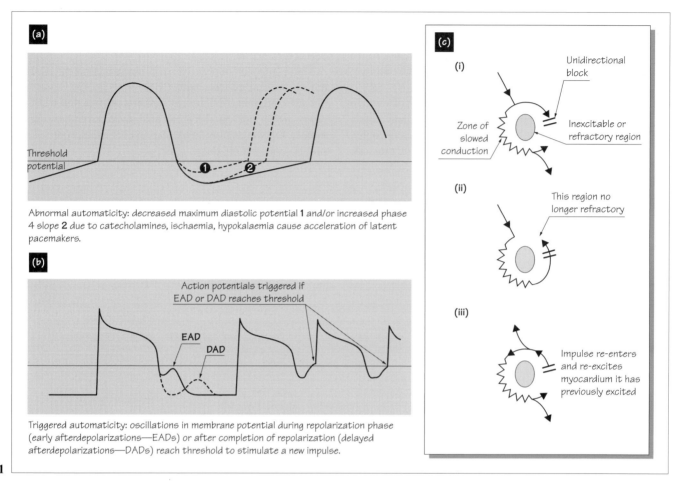

(a)

Threshold potential

① **②**

Abnormal automaticity: decreased maximum diastolic potential **1** and/or increased phase 4 slope **2** due to catecholamines, ischaemia, hypokalaemia cause acceleration of latent pacemakers.

(b)

Action potentials triggered if EAD or DAD reaches threshold

EAD
DAD

Triggered automaticity: oscillations in membrane potential during repolarization phase (early afterdepolarizations—EADs) or after completion of repolarization (delayed afterdepolarizations—DADs) reach threshold to stimulate a new impulse.

(c)

(i)
Unidirectional block
Zone of slowed conduction
Inexcitable or refractory region

(ii)
This region no longer refractory

(iii)
Impulse re-enters and re-excites myocardium it has previously excited

45.1

Arrhythmias are abnormalities of the heart rate or rhythm which can be caused by disorders of impulse **generation** (abnormal automaticity, triggered automaticity) or **conduction** (re-entry).

Abnormal automaticity

All parts of the conduction system demonstrate a spontaneous phase 4 depolarization and are potential or *latent* cardiac pacemakers. Because sinoatrial node (SAN) pacemaking is of the highest frequency (70–80 beats/min), it causes **overdrive suppression** of pacemaking by the atrioventricular node (AVN) (50–60 beats/min) or Purkinje fibres (30–40 beats/min). However, ischaemia, hypokalaemia, fibre stretch, or local catecholamine release can increase automaticity in these latent pacemakers (Fig. 45.1a), which can then override SA nodal pacemaking to cause arrhythmia.

Atrial and ventricular muscle cells normally do not demonstrate spontaneous activity. However, even these cells can develop repetitive impulse initiation and cause arrhythmias if the membrane potential is sufficiently depolarized. The reduction of membrane potential is usually a result of underlying cardiac disease, most commonly ischaemia. The threshold at which such **depolarization-induced automaticity** develops is quite variable. Automatic rhythms may demonstrate 'warm up' and 'cool down' phenomena, where the rate gradually accelerates to a constant level and then slows prior to termination of the arrhythmia.

Triggered automaticity

Triggered automaticity is caused by **afterdepolarizations**. These oscillations in the membrane potential occur during (**early afterdepolarizations**) or after (**delayed afterdepolarizations**) repolarization has occurred. Oscillations large enough to reach threshold initiate premature action potentials and heart beats. This may occur repeatedly, initiating a sustained arrhythmia (Fig. 45.1b) Afterdepolarization magnitude is influenced by changes in heart rate, catecholamines, and parasympathetic withdrawal.

Early afterdepolarizations (EADs) occur during the terminal plateau or repolarization phases of the action potential. They develop more readily in Purkinje fibres than in ventricular or atrial myocytes. EAD can be induced by agents that prolong action potential duration and increase the inward current (e.g. aconitine, a toxin from buttercups that prevents Na^+-channel inactivation). Blockade of K^+ currents can also cause EADs and triggered activity by increasing action potential duration and delaying repolarization. Drugs having this effect include sotalol, *n*-acetyl procainamide (a procainamide metabolite), and quinidine. These are most likely to cause EADs during hypokalaemia or when the heart rate is slow. The arrhythmias induced by drugs that cause EADs resemble a type of arrhythmia called **torsade de pointes**.

Delayed afterdepolarizations (DADs) are caused by an excessive increase in $[Ca^{2+}]_i$ in myocardial cells. The classical DAD-induced arrhythmia occurs with digitalis toxicity, which increases $[Ca^{2+}]_i$ by a mechanism described in Chapter 44. DADs can also be caused by catecholamines, which increase Ca^{2+} influx through the L-type Ca^{2+} channel. The **transient inward current** responsible for the oscillation of membrane potential following an increase in $[Ca^{2+}]_i$ appears to be caused by entry of Na^+. The occurrence and magnitude of DADs and the likelihood that they will cause arrhythmias is increased by conditions that enhance the transient inward current. These include longer action potentials, which cause larger increases in $[Ca^{2+}]_i$. Therefore drugs prolonging action potential duration may trigger DADs, whereas drugs shortening the action potential have the opposite effect. The magnitude of the transient inward current is also influenced by the resting membrane potential, and is maximal when this is approximately -60 mV.

Abnormal impulse conduction—re-entry

Re-entry occurs when an impulse that is delayed in one region of the heart re-excites adjacent areas of myocardium more than once (Fig. 45.1c). Emergence of re-entrant arrhythmias requires several conditions to be present:

1 There must be a *central inexcitable region*, around which the re-entrant impulse can circulate. This central obstacle may be anatomical (e.g. scar tissue) or functional, as in a region of cells which are refractory.

2 Impulse conduction should be delayed at some stage in the circuit to allow tissues in front of the impulse to recover from refractoriness. This is usually due to a zone of *slowed conduction*.

3 The circuit must also include a zone of *unidirectional block*, where conduction is blocked in one direction while remaining possible in the other.

For example, re-entry may occur when an impulse encounters a region of scar tissue, and is conducted slowly on one side, but is blocked unidirectionally on the other (Fig. 45.1c(i)). The slowed impulse can sweep around the inexcitable zone and traverse the region of unidirectional block in a retrograde direction. If the impulse has been delayed sufficiently, the myocardium on the other side is no longer refractory and the impulse *re-enters* and re-excites it (Fig. 45.1c(ii)). This impulse may continue to circle the central barrier. As long as this re-entrant circuit persists (anything from one cardiac cycle up to an indefinite period), it may give off impulses that are conducted to the rest of the heart to cause arrhythmia (Fig. 45.1c(iii)).

Slowed conduction occurs when the amplitude and slope of phase 0 depolarization are depressed, causing a diminution of axial current flow. *Depressed fast responses* occur when impulses arise in situations where many (but not all) Na^+ channels are inactivated, and therefore unable to open. This can happen if an impulse arises prematurely during the relative refractory period, and also where the resting potential is low (-60 to -70 mV), in which case many channels remain inactivated for an abnormally long time following action potentials. At membrane potential levels positive of -60 mV, Na^+ channels are completely inactivated, but L-type Ca^{2+} channels can still open, resulting in a slowly propagated action potential termed a *slow response*.

Unidirectional block may occur as a consequence of regional differences in the length of the refractory period. For example, premature impulses will be blocked in regions with the longest refractory period, but conducted in other regions. This mechanism is described in Chapter 15 with reference to **Wolff–Parkinson–White** or **pre-excitation** syndrome, a condition in which the heart has a congenital *accessory pathway* between an atrium and ventricle which remains refractory for longer than the normal pathway through the AVN.

Premature impulses can also undergo unidirectional block in regions where conduction is depressed by ischaemic damage. This is most likely to be the mechanism of ventricular tachycardias during and after myocardial infarction. These re-entrant circuits frequently originate in epicardial muscle at the edge of a transmural infarct, in which the fibres are arranged in fascicles (bundles). Impulse transmission parallel to the fascicles is rapid, whereas in the transverse direction, the conduction is slow and may form apparent block.

Proarrhythmia

Proarrhythmia refers to the tendency of antiarrhythmic drugs to cause arrhythmias. Proarrhythmia can occur with all antiarrhythmic agents, but is particularly problematical with class IC drugs, which can increase mortality by causing lethal ventricular arrhythmias. Proarrhythmia is mainly caused by two mechanisms. Firstly, class IA and III drugs increase action potential duration (APD, Q–T prolongation). This promotes the occurrence of early and delayed afterdepolarizations, causing triggered automaticity (see Chapter 45). The dangerous ventricular arrhythmia **torsades de pointes** may ensue. Secondly, pronounced depression of conduction, especially by class IC drugs, can cause re-entrant rhythms by creating areas of unidirectional conduction block.

46 Specific arrhythmias

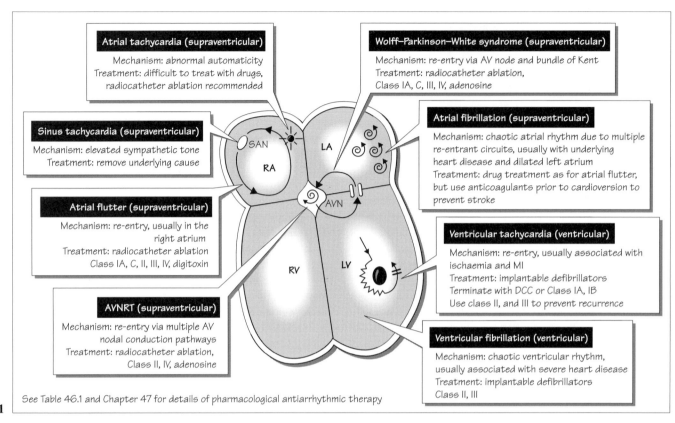

Atrial tachycardia (supraventricular)
Mechanism: abnormal automaticity
Treatment: difficult to treat with drugs,
radiocatheter ablation recommended

Wolff–Parkinson–White syndrome (supraventricular)
Mechanism: re-entry via AV node and bundle of Kent
Treatment: radiocatheter ablation,
Class IA, C, III, IV, adenosine

Sinus tachycardia (supraventricular)
Mechanism: elevated sympathetic tone
Treatment: remove underlying cause

Atrial fibrillation (supraventricular)
Mechanism: chaotic atrial rhythm due to multiple
re-entrant circuits, usually with underlying
heart disease and dilated left atrium
Treatment: drug treatment as for atrial flutter,
but use anticoagulants prior to cardioversion to
prevent stroke

Atrial flutter (supraventricular)
Mechanism: re-entry, usually in the
right atrium
Treatment: radiocatheter ablation
Class IA, C, II, III, IV, digitoxin

Ventricular tachycardia (ventricular)
Mechanism: re-entry, usually associated with
ischaemia and MI
Treatment: implantable defibrillators
Terminate with DCC or Class IA, IB
Use class II, and III to prevent recurrence

AVNRT (supraventricular)
Mechanism: re-entry via multiple AV
nodal conduction pathways
Treatment: radiocatheter ablation,
Class II, IV, adenosine

Ventricular fibrillation (ventricular)
Mechanism: chaotic ventricular rhythm,
usually associated with severe heart disease
Treatment: implantable defibrillators
Class II, III

SAN, RA, LA, AVN, RV, LV

See Table 46.1 and Chapter 47 for details of pharmacological antiarrhythmic therapy

46.1

The figure summarizes mechanisms and treatments for common arrhythmias. All of these (except ventricular fibrillation) cause tachycardia; bradyarrhythmias are described in Chapter 15.

Supraventricular tachycardias (SVT)

Supraventricular tachycardias are abnormalities in the timing or sequence of cardiac depolarization, originating at or above the atrioventricular node, which result in a heart rate of > 100 beats/min. These are usually troublesome rather than life threatening. Common symptoms include lightheadedness, palpitations, and shortness of breath. Rarely, sudden death can occur.

Sinus tachycardia (100–200 beats/min), the most common SVT, occurs when physiological (exercise) or pathological (phaeochromocytoma, congestive heart failure, thyrotoxicosis) stimuli elevate sympathetic tone, and accelerate SA nodal pacemaking. Sinus tachycardia generally starts and stops gradually. Treatment involves removing the underlying cause.

Atrial tachycardia is frequently caused by an abnormal (ectopic) pacemaker, and can occur in either atrium. Some atrial tachycardias are re-entrant in nature, frequently following surgery that involves incision into the atrium. The onset and offset of the tachycardia may be sudden or gradual.

Atrial flutter results from re-entry in an atrium (usually the right), with an area of slowed conduction near the orifice of the inferior vena cava and a circuit involving the whole atrium. The atrial rate is typically 300 beats/min, with a ventricular rate that is 150 (2 : 1), 100 (3 : 1) or 75 (4 : 1) per min depending on AVN conduction. Both atrial flutter and atrial fibrillation (see below) are typically seen in patients with underlying cardiac disease, often associated with atrial dilatation. These conditions are particularly common in older hypertensives, and may also be caused by acute pulmonary thromboembolism or thyrotoxicosis. However, both conditions can also develop paroxysmally in patients without underlying heart disease. Attempts to cardiovert (restore normal *sinus rhythm*) atrial flutter with class IA drugs (see Table 46.1) may cause severe ventricular tachycardia and sudden death by establishing 1 : 1 AV nodal conduction. This occurs because these drugs suppress vagal firing, thereby increasing AV nodal conduction. This hazard is avoided by preadministering a drug that suppresses AV nodal conduction (e.g. a β-blocker, digoxin).

Atrial fibrillation is a chaotic atrial rhythm resulting in an atrial rate of 350–600 beats/min and a lack of effective atrial contraction. The ventricular rate is typically less than 200 beats/min, because the AVN is unable to conduct most of the atrial

Table 46.1 The Vaughan Williams and Singh classification system of antiarrhythmic drugs.

Class/Mechanism	Major actions on atrial and ventricular myocardium	Major actions on nodal tissue	Use
IA: Block of Na+ channels (dissoc ~5 s)	Slow/depress conduction ↑ APD and ERP		SV and V tachycardias
IB: Block of Na+ channels (dissoc ~500 ms)	Slight ↓ of APD and ERP in normal tissue, but greatly slow/depress conduction and ↑ ERP in depolarized/rapidly firing tissue		V tachycardias esp. associated with AMI
IC: Block of Na+ channels (dissoc 10–20 s)	Strongly slow/depress conduction Little effect on APD and ERP ↓ contractility		Mainly life-threatening V tachycardias
II: Block of β-receptors	Abolish abnormal automaticity caused by increased symp. drive ↓ contractility	Inhibit SAN automaticity and ↑ ERP in AVN	V and SV tachycardias, esp. during and after AMI
III: Increased APD and ERP, usually block K+ channels	Greatly ↑ APD and ERP	Inhibit SAN automaticity and ↑ ERP in AVN	V and SV tachycardias
IV: Block of Ca²⁺ channels	↓ contractility and APD	↓ conduction velocity and ↑ ERP in AVN ↓ normal and abnormal automaticity in SAN and AVN	SV tachycardias

impulses impinging upon it. Studies suggest that this arrhythmia is caused by five to seven unstable re-entrant circuits with very short cycle lengths, which progress across the atrium, temporarily disappearing and then reforming. Palpitations, dyspnoea, presyncope or syncope may occur due to the increased ventricular rate or the absence of atrial systolic filling. Atrial fibrillation is a major cause of stroke. Thrombi form in the left atrial cavity or appendage because the lack of coordinated atrial contraction leads to stasis of blood. Thrombi may embolize to the systemic circulation, particularly the brain and limbs.

Ventricular arrhythmias

These arrhythmias are localized to the ventricles. The ECG demonstrates a rapid, broad complex rhythm, with a bizarre QRS complex. The atrial activity is often independent of ventricular rhythm. Patients usually have underlying structural heart disease, leading to a poor prognosis with 50% mortality at 2 years.

Sustained **ventricular tachycardia (VT)** is associated with MI, cardiomyopathy, and valvular and congenital heart disease. VT usually results from micro-re-entrant circuits occurring in the border zone of infarcted tissue, although the rhythm may be initiated by ventricular ectopic beats caused by an automatic or triggered automatic mechanism. The rhythm may cause haemodynamic collapse or degenerate into ventricular fibrillation. VT is uncommon in structurally normal hearts, but specific varieties are recognized, including right ventricular ouflow tract tachycardia and fascicular tachycardia.

Ventricular fibrillation (VF) is a chaotic ventricular rhythm causing an immediate loss of cardiac output and death unless the patient is resuscitated. VF is generally associated with severe underlying heart disease, including ischaemic heart disease and cardiomyopathy, but occurs occasionally in a normal heart (idiopathic VF). VF may follow episodes of VT or of acute ischaemia, and frequently causes sudden death during MI. Following one event, there is a high recurrence rate.

Nonpharmacogical treatments for arrhythmias

Direct current (DC) cardioversion allows rapid cardioversion of VF and haemodynamically unstable SVT and VT. Shocks of 50–360 J are delivered to the anaesthetized patient via paddles placed over the sternum and the right ventricular apex.

In **radiofrequency catheter ablation** the accessory pathways or focally automatic myocardium causing certain tachyarrhythmias is ablated by focal heating delivered via a catheter. The catheter is placed transvenously and the tip is located at the surface of the endocardium at the site of the abnormality. Radiofrequency energy is delivered to the catheter tip, and dissipated to a large indifferent plate, usually over the back. The tip temperature is set to 60–65°C, resulting in a lesion 8–10 mm in diameter and of a similar depth. This extremely safe and controllable technique is curative in > 90% of cases.

Implantable defibrillators consist of a generator connected to electrodes placed transvenously in the heart and superior vena cava. A sensing circuit detects arrhythmias, which are classified as tachycardia or fibrillation on the basis of rate. The treatment algorithm is either as burst pacing, which can terminate VT with a high degree of success, or by the delivery of a shock at up to 40 J, which can cardiovert VT and VF. Shock delivery is between an electrode in the right ventricle and another in the superior vena cava or to the body of the generator (active can). Refinements in detection allow distinction of supraventricular and ventricular arrhythmias, so that several tiers of progressively more aggressive therapy can be set up. The AVID study reported in 1997 that in patients with malignant ventricular arrhythmia, this approach improved survival by 31% over 3 years compared to antiarrhythmic drug therapy (mainly amiodarone).

47 Antiarrhythmic drugs

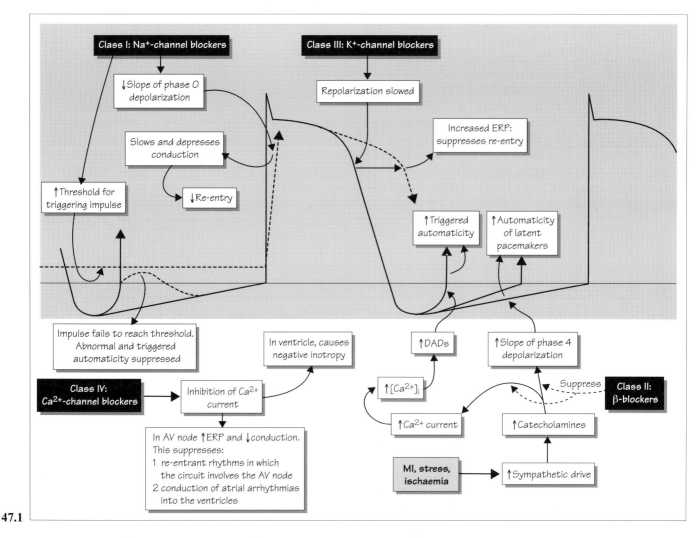

47.1

Most antiarrhythmic drugs, whatever their specific mechanisms, cause two useful actions which allow them to reduce abnormal electrical activity, while having tolerably small effects on normal myocardium:

1 They suppress abnormal (ectopic) pacemakers more than they do the sinoatrial node (SAN) pacemaker.
2 They increase the ratio of effective refractory period to action potential duration: ERP/APD.

The Vaughan Williams and Singh classification system (see Table 46.1) for antiarrhythmic drugs is used because it is relatively simple. However, it excludes several useful agents, and is not very useful for matching specific drugs to particular arrhythmias. Furthermore, *most antiarrhythmic drugs have properties of more than one class*. This often arises because the drugs exist as 50/50 mixtures of two stereo-isomers having nonidentical actions, or because drug metabolites have their own separate antiarrhythmic effects.

The **Sicilian gambit**, proposed in 1991, is a scheme designed to help match antiarrhythmic drugs to specific arrhythmias. It is based on identifying the characteristic of the arrhythmia that can be most easily corrected, and then selecting the drug that has the combination of actions most likely to target this characteristic.

Class I drugs (see also Table 46.1)

Class I drugs act primarily by blocking Na$^+$ channels. Although class I subtypes have somewhat different actions, all depress and slow conduction, especially in myocardium depolarized by ischaemia. Depression of conduction can interrupt re-entrant pathways by deepening a unidirectional block, thereby rendering it bidirectional. Class I drugs can also suppress automaticity (Fig. 47.1, upper left).

Na$^+$ channels are **closed** during diastole, and cycle through **open** and **inactivated** states during the cardiac action potential (see Chapter 10). Class I drugs have a higher affinity for open and/or inactivated Na^+ channels compared to closed channels. Consequently, they bind to Na^+ channels during each action potential and then progressively dissociate following repolarization. Channel block is therefore **use dependent** and **frequency dependent**, because drug bound to channels accumulates when opening ('use') is frequent. In addition, dissociation is slowed when the resting potential is depolarized.

Class IB drugs (**lidocaine, tocainide, mexilitine**) have little effect on normal myocardium, because they dissociate rapidly (< 500 ms) and therefore almost completely between action potentials. However, in tissue which is depolarized, or firing impulses at high frequency, dissociation between impulses is incomplete, and channel blockade occurs. Lidocaine is therefore useful in treating ventricular tachyarrhythmias associated with MI, which mainly originate in myocardium depolarized by ischaemia. Lidocaine is given intravenously because extensive first-pass metabolism occurs. Tocainide and mexilitine are similar to lidocaine in structure and action, but can be given orally.

Class IC drugs (**flecainide** and **propafenone**) have a less use-dependent action, because their dissociation rate is so slow (10–20 s) that they remain bound to channels from one action potential to the next, even at a low frequency of stimulation. They strongly depress conduction in both normal and depolarized myocardium. This is useful for blocking re-entrant pathways in which conduction is already weak, but also reduces contractility. These drugs are used for supraventricular arrhythmias, particularly Wolf–Parkinson–White syndrome, and to abolish acute ventricular tachycardias. **Moricizine** is a mixed class IB/IC agent.

Class IA drugs (**quinidine, procainamide**, and **disopyramide**) dissociate from the Na^+ channel at an intermediate rate (< 5 s), thereby lengthening the ERP. They also have class III activity, which prolongs APD. These drugs depress both conduction and abnormal pacemaker activity, therefore suppressing a wide range of ventricular and supraventricular arrhythmias. Quinidine and disopyramide have antimuscarinic effects, and often cause nausea, vomiting, and diarrhoea. Quinidine can also cause *chinconism* (tinnitus, dizziness, headache). Disopyramide reduces contractility, which may be dangerous if left ventricular dysfunction is present. Procainamide has weaker antimuscarinic and gastrointestinal effects, but chronic use can cause a lupus-like syndrome, especially in those who metabolize it slowly.

Class II drugs

Class II drugs are β-blockers. Catecholamine elevation associated with MI and heart failure stimulates cardiac β-receptors, causing arrhythmias through multiple mechanisms (Fig. 47.1, lower right). An increase in phase 4 depolarization may cause sinus tachycardia. Other normally latent cardiac pacemakers may become spontaneously active. Elevations in $[Ca^{2+}]_i$ due to enhanced Ca^{2+}-channel activation promote delayed afterdepolarizations. These effects are antagonized by β-blockers, including **propranolol, metoprolol, atenolol**, and **timolol**. At higher concentrations β-blockers block Na^+ channels, but this action is unlikely to contribute much to their therapeutic effect.

Class III drugs

Class III drugs increase APD and therefore prolong ERP. Re-entry occurs when an impulse is locally delayed, and then re-enters and re-excites adjacent myocardium (see Chapter 45). Drugs which prolong ERP prevent this re-excitation, because the adjacent myocardium is still refractory (inexcitable) at the time when the delayed impulse reaches it. The class III agents **amiodarone, sotalol** and **bretylium** increase APD by inhibiting K^+ channels and slowing repolarization. However, each drug has additional actions, which may be useful.

Amiodarone is effective against many supraventricular and ventricular arrhythmias, probably because it also has class Ia, II, and IV actions (it also blocks α-receptors!). Clinical trials show that amiodarone modestly reduces mortality after MI and in congestive heart failure. However, its long-term use is recommended only if other antiarrhythmic drugs fail, because it has many cumulative adverse effects and must be discontinued in about a third of patients. Hazards include pulmonary fibrosis, hypo- and hyperthyroidism, liver dysfunction, photosensitivity, and peripheral neuropathy. Amiodarone also has a very unpredictable and long (4–15 weeks) plasma half-life, which complicates its oral administration. Sotalol is a mixed class II and III drug used for ventricular and supraventricular arrhythmias. Although it causes far fewer side effects than amiodarone, it is more likely to cause torsades de pointes.

Class IV drugs

Class IV drugs (**verapamil** and **diltiazem**) exert their antiarrhythmic effects on the atrioventricular node (AVN), by blocking L-type Ca^{2+} channels mediating the nodal action potential. Effects on AVN electrical activity include slowing of depolarization, an increased refractory period, and slowing of AV conduction. Ca^{2+}-channel blockade is use dependent, and AV block is enhanced by cell depolarization and high-frequency firing. These drugs are used mainly to treat supraventricular tachycardias. They suppress AV nodal re-entrant rhythms by depressing conduction. They can slow the ventricular rate in atrial flutter and fibrillation by preventing a proportion of atrial impulses from being conducted through the AVN. Negative inotropy can occur due to L-type channel inhibition, especially if left ventricular function is impaired. Negative inotropic and chronotropic effects are exacerbated by coadministration of β-blockers.

Adenosine, an endogenous nucleoside (Chapters 22, 24), acts on myocardial A_1-receptors, suppressing the Ca^{2+} current and enhancing K^+ currents. These effects depress AV nodal conduction. Adenosine is the drug of choice for rapid termination of many supraventricular tachycardias. It commonly causes transient flushing and breathlessness. **Digoxin** slows AV conduction by stimulating the vagus and is used to slow atrial fibrillation and other supraventricular tachycardias, especially in patients with heart failure (see Chapter 44).

48 Diseases of the aortic valve

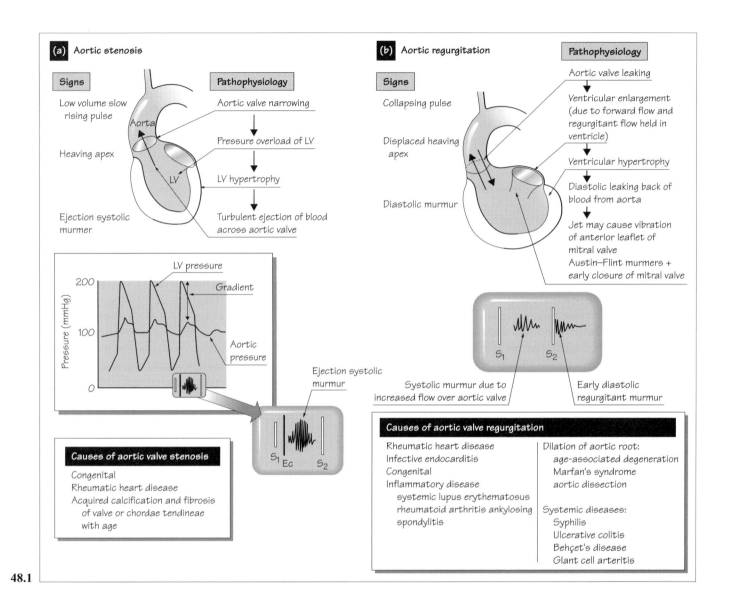

(a) Aortic stenosis

Signs
- Low volume slow rising pulse
- Heaving apex
- Ejection systolic murmer

Pathophysiology
- Aortic valve narrowing
  ↓
- Pressure overload of LV
  ↓
- LV hypertrophy
  ↓
- Turbulent ejection of blood across aortic valve

Aorta
LV

LV pressure
Gradient
Aortic pressure

Ejection systolic murmur

S_1 Ec S_2

Causes of aortic valve stenosis
- Congenital
- Rheumatic heart disease
- Acquired calcification and fibrosis of valve or chordae tendineae with age

(b) Aortic regurgitation

Signs
- Collapsing pulse
- Displaced heaving apex
- Diastolic murmur

Pathophysiology
- Aortic valve leaking
- Ventricular enlargement (due to forward flow and regurgitant flow held in ventricle)
- Ventricular hypertrophy
  ↓
- Diastolic leaking back of blood from aorta
- Jet may cause vibration of anterior leaflet of mitral valve
- Austin–Flint murmers + early closure of mitral valve

S_1 S_2

Systolic murmur due to increased flow over aortic valve

Early diastolic regurgitant murmur

Causes of aortic valve regurgitation

Rheumatic heart disease	Dilation of aortic root:
Infective endocarditis	age-associated degeneration
Congenital	Marfan's syndrome
Inflammatory disease	aortic dissection
systemic lupus erythematosus	
rheumatoid arthritis ankylosing	Systemic diseases:
spondylitis	Syphilis
	Ulcerative colitis
	Behçet's disease
	Giant cell arteritis

48.1

The **aortic valve** is normally tricuspid and separates the left ventricle (LV) from the aorta. Impaired aortic valve opening (**aortic stenosis**, AS) impedes outflow of blood and imposes a pressure load on the LV. Deficient valve closure (**aortic regurgitation**, AR, *incompetence*) allows blood to flow back from the aorta, and imposes a volume load on the LV.

Aortic stenosis
Causes
Acquired calcific aortic stenosis is the most common cause. Calcium deposits occur at the base of the cusp, without involvement of the commissures. This is most likely related to prolonged mechanical stress, and is more common in people with congenital bicuspid valves. About 50% of patients < 70 years old with significant AS have bicuspid valves, whereas most old patients with AS have tricuspid valves. ***Rheumatic***: AS as a result of rheumatic heart disease is unusual without coexisting mitral valve disease. Male sex, diabetes and hypercholesterolaemia are also risk factors for AS.

Congenital
A **unicuspid aortic valve** is usually fatal within 1 year from birth. **Bicuspid** aortic valves develop progressive fusion of the commissures and symptoms usually present after 40 years. Infants with atherosclerosis due to lipid disorders may develop AS in conjunction with **coronary artery disease** (CAD).

Pathophysiology

A slow reduction of aortic valve area causes **left ventricular hypertrophy** and eventual myocardial dysfunction, arrhythmias, and **left heart failure** (see Chapter 43). 'Critical' AS occurs with > 75% reduction of valve area to < 0.5 cm^2/m^2 body surface area, and a > 50 mmHg gradient between peak systolic LV and aortic pressure at a normal cardiac output. With worsening AS, cardiac output cannot increase adequately during exercise and eventually becomes insufficient at rest. At this point the LV dilates, and left ventricular EDP increases to the point where overt LV failure ensues.

Clinical features

Patients present usually between the ages of 50 and 70 years, most commonly with **angina** (50% have concurrent CAD). Angina is due to the increased oxygen needs of the hypertrophied LV and inadequate cardiac output during exercise. Exercise tolerance is decreased, and if brain bloodflow is insufficient patients may develop **exercise-associated syncope**. Once patients with AS develop angina, syncope or LV failure, their median survival is < 3 years.

Patients with mild AS have a normal blood pressure and pulse. In moderate to severe AS there is a slow-rising, low-volume pulse that may demonstrate a **thrill** (vibration) and decreased pulse pressure. Auscultation reveals a normal S$_1$, a single S$_2$ because of an absent aortic component, a S$_4$, and a harsh late **systolic murmur**, preceded by an ejection click (Ec) (see Fig. 48.1a and Chapter 13), heard best in the right second intercostal space and transmitted to the carotids and apex. It is louder with squatting and softer with standing or during the **Valsalva manoeuvre** (forced expiration against a closed glottis). With worsening AS and a fall in cardiac output, the murmur may become softer (**silent AS**).

Investigations

The ECG shows LV hypertrophy with strain (depressed ST, inverted T), and left atrial delay. Atrial fibrillation and ventricular arrhythmias are often seen when LV function has deteriorated. Echocardiography shows reduced valve opening, calcification of cusps, and allows calculation of valve area. Doppler imaging allows calculation of the pressure gradient between the LV and aorta.

Management

It is important that systemic hypotension and arterial vasodilatation be avoided. β-adrenergic blockers and other negative inotropic agents should thus not be used. Once symptoms develop, cardiac catheterization with **coronary angiography** must be performed prior to valve replacement, and coronary artery bypass performed if significant CAD is present. Several types of mechanical valve are available, including those of a 'ball and cage' variety or tilting disk. These will always require **anticoagulant therapy**. Valves can also be obtained from pigs or human cadavers and these have the advantage that anticoagulants are not generally required. **Balloon valvuloplasty** can be performed in children with noncalcified valves, but is of little value in adults.

Aortic regurgitation

Causes

Causes of aortic regurgitation (AR) include **rheumatic disease**, where fibrous retraction of the valve cusps prevents apposition, **infective endocarditis** causing valve damage and **congenital malformations** (e.g. bicuspid valve) (see Fig. 48.1, right).

Pathophysiology

AR imposes a volume load on the LV because of flow back into the ventricle. **Acute AR** (trauma, infective endocarditis, aortic dissection) is usually catastrophic. Here the LV cannot accommodate the acute increase in volume and LVEDP rises. The early increase in LVEDP causes premature closure of the mitral valve and inadequate forward LV filling, resulting in cardiovascular collapse and acute respiratory failure.

In **chronic AR**, volume load and LVEDP increase gradually, and **LV hypertrophy** allows adequate output to be maintained. As the aortic valve never completely closes, there is no LV isovolumetric relaxation phase (see Chapter 13) and the pulse pressure is wide. Cardiac output is aided by a baroreceptor-mediated fall in afterload.

Clinical features

Patients usually do not present with symptoms until LV failure develops. Signs include a wide pulse pressure (caused by reduction in diastolic pressure) and a **collapsing pulse** (Chapter 13). This may occasionally cause visible nail bed pulsation and pulsatile head bobbing. The LV apex is displaced laterally and is hyperdynamic. Auscultation reveals a high-pitched **early diastolic murmur** at the left sternal border, and a **systolic flow murmur** across the aortic valve. A low-frequency **rumbling late diastolic murmur** at the apex (**Austin–Flint murmur**) may be caused by premature closing of the mitral valve.

Investigations

Echocardiography can determine the aetiology and severity of AR by imaging the valve leaflets and LV dimensions, aortic root diameter, and diastolic closure or fluttering of the mitral valve. Doppler imaging quantifies the amount of regurgitation flow.

Management

Acute severe AR requires urgent valve replacement. Chronic AR has a generally good prognosis until symptoms develop. Patients with moderate AR should be followed with serial echocardiography. Valve replacement should be considered in patients with symptoms, or in asymptomatic patients with worsening LV dimensions, LV function, or aortic root diameter. Valve replacement is similar to that for aortic stenosis, except that replacement of the aortic root may also be required in patients with a severely dilated ascending aorta.

49 Diseases of the mitral valve

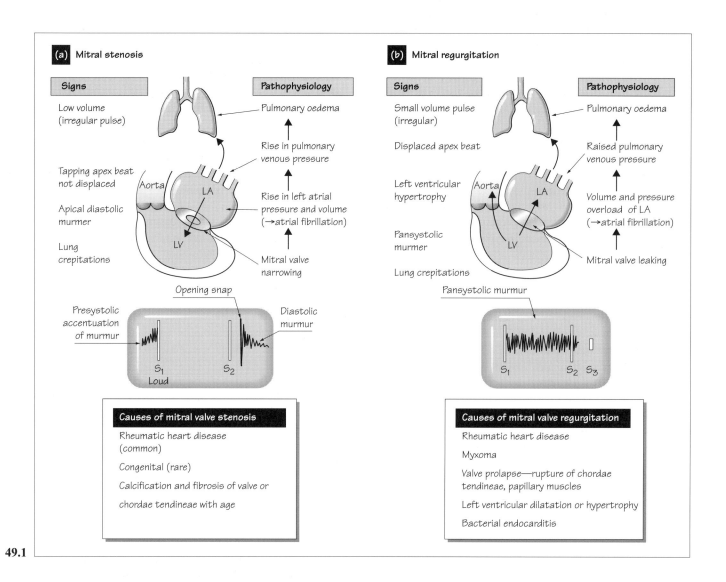

The **mitral valve** is normally bicuspid and separates the left atrium (LA) and left ventricle (LV). The valve may narrow (**mitral stenosis**) or leak (**mitral regurgitation**).

Mitral stenosis
Causes
Mitral stenosis (MS) is usually due to prior episodes of acute **rheumatic fever**. This causes thickening and fusion of the mitral **commissures**, **cusps**, or **chordae tendineae**, making the cusps less flexible and narrowing the orifice. Symptoms from MS usually develop > 10 years after the acute attack, which patients may not recall. The normal area of a mitral valve is 6 cm²; critical MS occurs when this area falls to 1 cm².

Pathophysiology
Mitral stenosis prevents the free flow of blood from the LA to the LV, and slows ventricular filling during diastole. The left atrial pressure rises to maintain cardiac output, and there is **atrial hypertrophy** and **dilatation**. The elevated left atrial pressure causes pulmonary congestion and can result in **pulmonary hypertension** and **oedema**, and **right heart failure** (see Chapter 43). Patients with MS rely on atrial systole for ventricular filling, and **atrial fibrillation** (caused by atrial enlargement) significantly reduces cardiac output. The fibrillating atrium is liable to develop **thrombi** that may be **embolized** (dislodge and move freely in the blood) causing stroke. The LV is usually normal in MS, but may be abnormal due to either chronic under-feeding of the LV or rheumatic scarring.

Clinical features

Patients present in their 20–30s with **dyspnoea** on exertion or conditions that raise cardiac output (e.g. fever, pregnancy). This is a result of **pulmonary congestion**, which causes the lungs to become stiffer. Patients may present with **haemoptysis** (coughing up of blood), **palpitations**, or **stroke** (via embolization of thrombi). Symptoms may be precipitated by arrhythmias such as atrial fibrillation. Auscultation reveals an **opening snap** (OS) soon after S_2 that is heard best at the apex, and by a **rumbling diastolic murmur** leading to a loud S_1. The duration of the murmur is related to the severity of the MS. It is brief in mild MS and **holodiastolic** (*pandiastolic*, i.e. over the whole diastolic period) in severe MS. Patients in sinus rhythm may have **presystolic accentuation** of the murmur due to atrial contraction, and a large venous 'a' wave (see Chapter 13). If the mitral valve is completely immobile there may be no OS or a loud S_1. As MS becomes more severe, there will be a less prominent arterial pulse, **lung crackles** (*crepitations*; audible crackles because of fluid in the lungs), and elevation of the **jugular venous pressure**.

The ECG may show only LA enlargement, although many patients are in atrial fibrillation. The chest radiograph may show left atrial enlargement with normal left ventricular size, but with increasing severity of MS there may be pulmonary vascular congestion, enlarged pulmonary arteries, and right ventricular enlargement.

Management

Mild MS may require little treatment, although management should include avoidance of **anaemia** and **tachyarrhythmias** as these may precipitate decompensation and cardiac failure (see Chapter 43). Prophylactic antibiotics for **endocarditis** should be administered before invasive procedures and patients in atrial fibrillation should receive **anticoagulation** to decrease the occurrence of stroke. Patients with MS can remain minimally symptomatic for many years, but deteriorate quickly once symptoms begin to worsen. Therefore, **valve replacement** with a mechanical valve, **valvotomy** (surgical separation of commissures) or **balloon valvuloplasty** (use of a balloon catheter to force open cusps) should be performed in moderately symptomatic patients with a mitral valve area < 1.7 cm².

Mitral regurgitation
Causes

Acute mitral regurgitation (MR) is usually a result of **bacterial endocarditis**, **ruptured chordae tendineae**, or ischaemic **papillary muscle rupture**. Chronic MR is now most likely to arise from **myxomatous degeneration** of the mitral leaflets or **valve prolapse** (reversal into atrium). Chronic MR may also develop in any disease causing LV dilatation, so preventing apposition (coming together) of the mitral leaflets, or because of ischaemic dysfunction of the papillary muscles.

Pathophysiology

In **acute MR** the LV ejects blood back into the LA, imposing a sudden volume load on the LA during ventricular systole. Left atrial pressure rises suddenly and this is rapidly followed by a rise in pulmonary venous pressure and capillary pressure. **Pulmonary oedema** ensues as a result of alteration of haemodynamics across the pulmonary vascular bed.

Chronic MR is sufficiently slow to allow compensatory LV dilatation and hypertrophy, and dilatation of the LA. The latter protects the pulmonary circulation from the effects of the regurgitant volume. MR imposes a diastolic volume load on the LV that causes dilatation, because each systolic stroke volume is composed of a portion that enters the aorta (LV output) and an ineffective portion that re-enters the LA (LV regurgitant volume) and adds to the venous return. The regurgitant volume increases when LV emptying is impaired, such as with aortic stenosis or hypertension.

Clinical features

Patients with mild chronic MR are usually asymptomatic. As MR worsens, patients develop **fatigue, dyspnoea on exertion, orthopnoea** and **pulmonary oedema** as a result of progressive LV failure and elevation of pulmonary capillary pressure (see Chapter 43). The development of atrial fibrillation is common because of dilatation of the LA. Chronic MR is associated with a **holosystolic** murmur which is heard best at the apex, with transmission to the axilla and the left infrascapular region. S_1 is soft and S_2 is split widely because of an early aortic component. Echocardiography can detect a prolapsing or rheumatic valve, and determine LV size and function. Doppler imaging of the regurgitant jet can assess the severity of MR.

Management

Management is focused on promoting LV emptying into the aorta. Reduction of afterload with **ACE inhibitors** is beneficial (see Chapter 44). Patients with atrial fibrillation receive **anticoagulants** to prevent stroke. A prolapsing valve may sometimes be repaired. Dilatation of the mitral valve ring may be corrected by implantation of an artificial ring. Rheumatic valves and those damaged by endocarditis often need replacement with an artificial valve. Valve replacement is best performed prior to the development of LV dysfunction or chronic pulmonary hypertension, and should always be performed in patients with symptomatic MR despite medical therapy. The risks of surgery are higher in acute MR; however, valve replacement should be performed in patients with uncontrollable heart failure or end-organ failure, even in cases of acute infective endocarditis.

50 Congenital heart disease

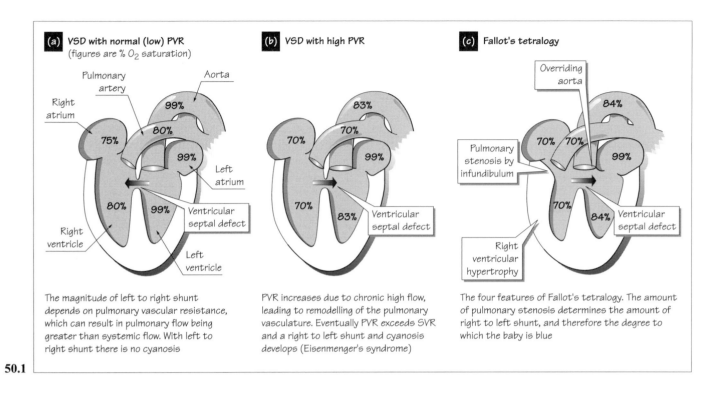

(a) VSD with normal (low) PVR (figures are % O_2 saturation)

Pulmonary artery · Aorta · Right atrium · 99% · 80% · 75% · 99% · Left atrium · 80% · 99% · Ventricular septal defect · Right ventricle · Left ventricle

The magnitude of left to right shunt depends on pulmonary vascular resistance, which can result in pulmonary flow being greater than systemic flow. With left to right shunt there is no cyanosis

(b) VSD with high PVR

83% · 70% · 70% · 99% · 70% · 83% · Ventricular septal defect

PVR increases due to chronic high flow, leading to remodelling of the pulmonary vasculature. Eventually PVR exceeds SVR and a right to left shunt and cyanosis develops (Eisenmenger's syndrome)

(c) Fallot's tetralogy

Overriding aorta · 84% · Pulmonary stenosis by infundibulum · 70% · 70% · 99% · 70% · 84% · Ventricular septal defect · Right ventricular hypertrophy

The four features of Fallot's tetralogy. The amount of pulmonary stenosis determines the amount of right to left shunt, and therefore the degree to which the baby is blue

50.1

Definition
Congenital heart diseases (CHDs) are abnormalities of cardiac structure that are present from birth. They result from abnormalities in cardiac development occurring between 3 and 8 weeks of gestation.

Incidence
The incidence of CHD is ~1% of live births, not including congenital valve disorders such as mitral prolapse or bicuspid aortic valve. Many spontaneous abortions or stillborns have cardiac malformations, or chromosomal abnormalities associated with structural heart defects. Maternal factors such as **rubella infection**, alcohol abuse and some medications are associated with CHD.

Physiology
In the normal fetal circulation (see Chapter 25) blood crosses the **foramen ovale** from the right to the left atrium. Most of the blood ejected by the right ventricle enters the aorta via the **ductus arteriosis**, because pulmonary vascular resistance (PVR) is higher than systemic vascular resistance (SVR). After birth PVR falls to one-tenth of SVR, allowing bloodflow from the right ventricle through the lungs. Closure of the foramen ovale and ductus arteriosis establishes the adult circulations in series.

Clinical features
CHDs normally present in infancy with either **congestive heart failure** or **central cyanosis**. Congestive heart failure in an infant is usually due to a left to right shunt, such as a **ventricular septal defect** or a **patent ductus arteriosis** (PDA), or as a result of aortic coarctation or stenosis. Infants with congestive heart failure fail to thrive, and demonstrate symptoms similar to those in adults (see Chapter 43). **Central cyanosis**, blueness of the trunk and mucous membranes, is due to > 3–5 g/dl of deoxygenated haemoglobin in the arterial circulation. Central cyanosis may result from severe pulmonary disease, and intrapulmonary right to left shunt (arteriovenous malformation, AVM) or extrapulmonary right to left shunting. It is characteristic of **transposition of the great vessels** and **tetralogy of Fallot**.

Ventricular septal defect
This is the most common CHD, and may occur in isolation or with other abnormalities. Flow across the defect is determined by the relationship between the resistances of the pulmonary and systemic circulations. *In utero*, when PVR > SVR, most blood exits the left ventricle via the aorta. However, after birth PVR < SVR, and blood is shunted from the left to the right ventricle, and into the pulmonary artery (Fig. 50.1a). The magnitude of the shunt is related to the size of the defect as well as the relative sizes of PVR and SVR.

Clinical features

Ventricular septal defects (VSDs) should be suspected in an infant who fails to gain weight, and has frequent respiratory difficulties or infections. The VSD is diagnosed by a harsh systolic murmur at the left sternal border. In young children a moderate VSD may cause exercise limitation or fatigue, an enlarged heart, and biventricular hypertrophy. Echocardiography with Doppler imaging allows estimation of the size and location of the VSD. Shunting of blood from the left ventricle into the pulmonary circulation leads to pulmonary hypertension, which if persistent causes irreversible **pulmonary vascular remodelling**. Once PVR exceeds SVR the direction of the shunt reverses and cyanosis develops (Fig. 50.1b; **Eisenmenger's syndrome**). At this point surgical correction is not possible, and therefore infants with a significant VSD benefit from early surgery. In the case of smaller VSDs, 50% close spontaneously within 3–4 years. Children with VSDs have an increased risk of endocarditis and should receive prophylactic antibiotics before dental procedures.

Transposition of the great arteries

Transposition of the great arteries occurs when the left ventricle empties into the pulmonary artery and the right ventricle empties into the aorta. This may be associated with VSD, atrial septal defect (ASD), or PDA. The transposition results in two parallel circulations, where deoxygenated systemic venous blood is returned to the body and oxygenated pulmonary venous blood returns to the lungs. This causes severe central cyanosis. Unless corrected, this defect is fatal in one-third of cases within 2 weeks and in 90% of cases within a year. Surgical correction involves an arterial switch where the great vessels are transected and connected to their appropriate ventricles. Prior to surgery infants can be stabilized by the creation of an ASD with a catheter, which allows mixing of blood in the atria and oxygenation of systemic blood. Administration of PGE_1 delays closure of the ductus arteriosus and allows further access of oxygenated blood to the systemic circulation.

Fallot's tetralogy

This is the most common cyanotic CHD found in children surviving to 1 year (Fig. 50.1c). It consists of a VSD, pulmonary stenosis, an overriding aorta (positioning of the aorta over the VSD), and right ventricular hypertrophy. These lead to a high right ventricular pressure and right to left shunt. The degree of cyanosis depends on the pulmonary stenosis, which is usually a combination of infundibular stenosis and obstruction of the pulmonary valve. The subvalvular stenosis is caused by misalignment of the infundibular septum; when the latter contracts it may exacerbate the stenosis.

Clinical features

Infants with Fallot's tetralogy are slow to develop, and may present with dyspnoea, fatigue, and hypoxic episodes (**Fallot's or tetralogy spells**), characterized by rapidly worsening cyanosis, progressing to limpness, stroke, and loss of consciousness. There is usually a palpable RV impulse and a thrill at the left sternal border. There is no pulmonary component to the second heart sound, and a systolic ejection murmur which is inversely proportional to the degree of pulmonary stenosis. Surgical correction of the VSD and ventricular obstruction is performed in infancy and has < 5% mortality.

Atrial septal defects

These defects usually go unrecognized until adulthood. They generally involve the mid-septum in the ostium secundum and are distinct from a patent foramen ovale. The left to right shunt increases pulmonary bloodflow, which if sustained into adulthood leads to pulmonary vascular remodelling and fixed pulmonary hypertension. Adults with ASDs may also present with atrial arrhythmias or left ventricular failure. Once severe pulmonary hypertension develops, there may be reversal of the left to right shunt, and cyanosis due to right to left shunt.

Clinical features

There is normally a pulmonary ejection murmur, a wide fixed split S_2, and elevated jugular venous pressure. As pulmonary hypertension worsens, the murmur becomes softer and S_2 becomes louder. If discovered early, ASDs with significant left to right shunts should be repaired to prevent the development of irreversible pulmonary hypertension. Once a right to left shunt has developed, surgical repair of an ASD is not performed.

51 Cardiac transplantation

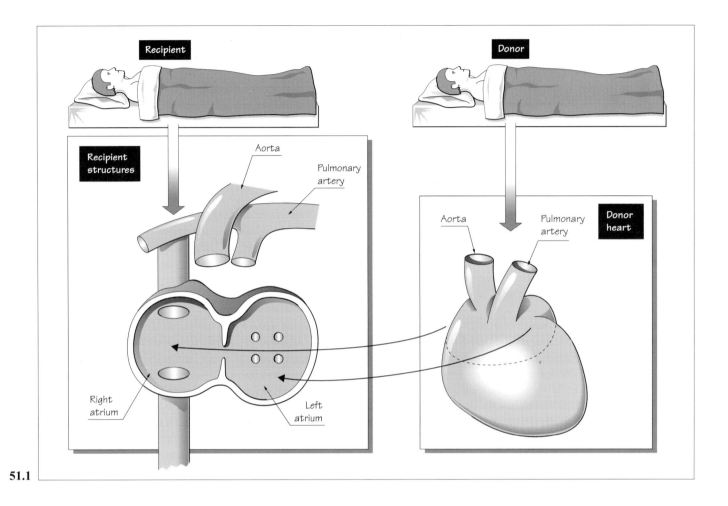

51.1

Definition
The explantation of the heart from a **brain-dead donor**, and implantation into a patient with **end-stage heart disease**. Cardiac transplantation is now a viable option for selected patients with irreversible severe cardiac disease. Over 30 000 cardiac transplants have been performed throughout the world.

Indications
Candidates should have severe cardiac disease refractory to medical or surgical treatment. Most patients have coronary artery disease or idiopathic cardiomyopathy as the underlying diagnosis.

Contraindications
Concurrent irreversible primary or secondary (e.g. due to diabetes) liver, kidney or lung disease, significant peripheral vascular or cerebrovascular disease, recent cancer, poor medical compliance, or severe immobility. Patients with pulmonary hypertension are at higher risk of postoperative acute right heart failure and may need to be considered for heart–lung transplantation. The upper age limit for eligibility is controversial. Most units have an age ceiling of 60–70 years with some variability based on the patient's overall health, underlying disease, and concurrent illnesses.

Recipients
The lack of donors means that ~25% of patients awaiting cardiac transplantation do not survive to surgery. They may require prolonged hospitalization and treatment with positive inotropic drugs (see Chapter 14). Left ventricular mechanical assist devices have been used as a bridge to transplantation. However, implantable mechanical hearts impart a poor prognosis to subsequent cardiac transplantation.

Donors
Potential heart donors should be **brain dead, normothermic**, and not receiving drugs such as hypnotics or paralytics. There should be no history of significant cardiac disease or malig-

nancy. There is no fixed upper age limit for donors, although angiography is often performed on older donors to determine the absence of significant coronary artery disease. The donor should have negative serology for HIV. The donor heart is preserved by flushing with cold **cardioplegia** (heart-paralysing) solution and external cooling. Ischaemic times of up to 6 h are not usually associated with significant post-transplant dysfunction. Matching of the donor heart to the recipient is by ABO blood grouping and size. Tissue matching is time consuming and only employed when the recipient has a high reactivity in a plasma-reactive antibody screen.

Surgery

The donor heart is anastomosed to a portion of the native posterior wall of the right and left atria with end-to-end anastomosis of the pulmonary artery and the aorta. This, however, results in a lack of coordination between atrial systole and ventricular filling, and distortion of the mitral and tricuspid valve annuli. The technique is therefore sometimes modified by creating venous anastomoses at the vena cavae and at the pulmonary veins. Methylprednisolone is often administered during surgery to prevent hyperacute rejection.

Aggressive **immunosuppression** is started immediately after surgery to limit acute rejection, usually with cyclosporin A or tacrolimus, plus prednisone and azathioprine. Monoclonal antibodies directed against CD3-positive lymphocytes may be used to prevent acute rejection.

Postoperative follow-up

Lifelong immune suppression usually consists of **cyclosporin A** or tacrolimus, **azathioprine** and **prednisone**. The need to prevent rejection must be balanced with the infectious complications of chronic immunosuppression. Acute rejection is monitored by transvenous endomyocardial biopsy and is most frequent in the first 3–6 months post-transplant. Biopsies are obtained from the right ventricular septum by passing a biopsy forceps into the heart from the internal jugular vein. Endomyocardial biopsy is performed periodically throughout the patient's life or if indicated by altered symptoms. Biopsies are graded on the severity of acute rejection based on the degree of lymphocytic infiltration, myocyte damage, or necrosis.

Episodes of acute rejection are generally treated with increased doses of corticosteroids, although antilymphocyte therapies may be necessary for refractory or severe episodes. The impact of newer generations of immunosuppressives such as **mycophenolate** or **rapamycin** on the development of acute rejection remains to be tested.

Most transplant patients develop at least one infection within the first year. In the first month post-transplantation most infections are caused by bacteria, which cause **nosocomial** (hospital-acquired) infection and present as **pneumonia**, **wound infection**, or catheter-related sepsis. Thereafter opportunistic infections,

most commonly **cytomegalovirus** (CMV), become more frequent, the risk being related to the degree of immunosuppression. CMV seronegative patients receiving a CMV seropositive heart have the greatest risk of developing CMV pneumonia, viraemia, hepatitis, gastritis, oesophagitis, or retinitis. However, CMV positive recipients are also at risk. The most lethal form of CMV infection is pneumonia, with a 10–20% mortality even with treatment using gancyclovir or foscarnet. Concurrent administration of CMV hyperimmune globulin may improve outcomes. The recent development of a PCR assay for CMV antigen has aided early detection of virus and may be useful in predicting patients who are at high risk. Most units administer CMV prophylaxis with gancyclovir or hyperimmune globulin in patients who are either seropositive prior to transplant or who receive a seropositive heart.

Other late opportunistic infections that occur commonly in the first year include **pneumocystis**, other fungi including **candida** and **aspergillus**, **nocardia**, **toxoplasmosis**, and **herpes simplex virus**. Routine use of prophylactic drug therapy has decreased the frequency of *Pneumocystis carinii* **pneumonia** and **toxoplasmosis**.

Late complications

After the first year opportunistic infections become less common, and complications as a result of drug treatment and graft atherosclerosis are more frequent causes of morbidity and mortality. Common drug complications include renal toxicity from cyclosporin or tacrolimus, and problems resulting from chronic administration of high doses of corticosteroids. These problems include osteoporosis, diabetes, cataracts, skin changes, lipid abnormalities, and psychiatric changes.

Graft atherosclerosis, a dreaded but common complication of cardiac transplantation, is distinct from typical atherosclerotic disease. It is characterized by intimal hyperplasia and smooth muscle hypertrophy in the graft vasculature, but without significant calcification. Patients with CMV infection have a higher frequency of developing graft atherosclerosis. Generally the lesions of graft atherosclerosis are diffuse and are not amenable to angioplasty or bypass grafting. Patients with severe disease have been re-transplanted, although the prognosis for the second transplantation is not as favourable as for the first.

Prognosis

Overall survival from cardiac transplantation is > 80% at 1 year and 60% at 5 years. Of the survivors, > 85% have significant improvement in lifestyle as assessed by performance status or quality of life. Approximately 50% of patients will go back to work. One-year survival for patients requiring re-transplantation (usually for graft atherosclerosis or severe acute rejection) is only 50–60%, with the difference likely to be related to the comorbidities that develop after the initial transplant.

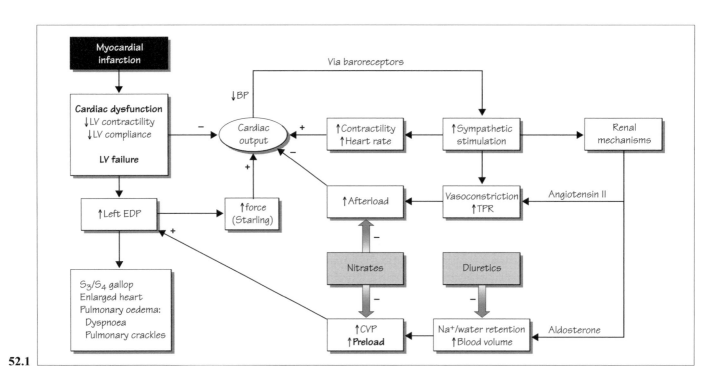

52.1

A 62-year-old man is transferred to your hospital because of recurrent chest pain and dyspnoea 5 days after suffering a large myocardial infarction. On the day of arrival he is free of chest pain but is still breathing with moderate difficulty. You obtain a chest radiograph, which confirms increased distended pulmonary vasculature, septal lines, and an enlarged heart. An echocardiogram shows an enlarged heart and an ejection fraction of 30% with minimal systolic motion of the anterior and apical portions of the heart. The patient is in normal sinus rhythm, with a heart rate of 110. Arterial blood pressure is 96/68, mean 82, respiratory rate 25/min. On cardiac auscultation you hear a S_3 gallop, a S_4 gallop, a normal S_1 and S_2, and a soft murmur that encompasses systole (holosystolic), and has uniform intensity that is heard at the apex and radiates to the left axilla. There are fine, late-inspiratory crackles (crepitations) heard about a third of the way up both lung fields. Arterial blood gases reveal a Pao_2 of 60 mmHg, $Paco_2$ of 30 mmHg, and pH of 7.37.

Questions

1 What is the left ventricular end-diastolic pressure likely to be in this patient and why?
2 What is the significance of the S_3 and S_4 gallop sounds?
3 Why is heart rate likely to be increased?
4 The arterial pressures are low. What is the peripheral vascular resistance likely to be in this case? What is the preload volume likely to be? How would similar arterial and venous loads probably affect arterial pressure in a normal heart?

5 You place a right heart catheter to assess the haemodynamics better, and find that the cardiac output is 3.0 L/min, and the right atrial pressure had a mean value of 10 mmHg. What is systemic vascular resistance? Is this normal?
6 How do abnormalities in contractile function, preload and afterload resistance play a role in this patient's current problem?
7 What might happen to cardiac output and arterial blood pressure if an arterial vasodilator was administered to this patient?
8 Would it be useful to alter contractility? In what direction? What might be a potential disadvantage of increasing contractility in this particular patient?
9 Suppose the arterial perfusion pressure during diastole could be increased while at the same time lowering it during systole. Would this intervention be useful? Why?

Answers

1 The left ventricular diastolic pressure is likely to be elevated. The recent myocardial infarction has diminished the pumping capacity of the ventricle, and to compensate the heart has filled to a larger diastolic volume to partially restore cardiac output and arterial pressures. The elevated cardiac filling pressures are reflected in the pulmonary venous pressures, and this has contributed to the pulmonary oedema. Cardiac enlargement is evident on the chest X-ray as an increase in heart size. The crackles are consistent with increased pulmonary interstitial and alveolar oedema.

2 The S_3 gallop is associated with early diastolic filling and is an indication of increased chamber stiffness. The S_4 gallop is associated with atrial contraction—late diastolic filling—and is associated with elevation of the end-diastolic pressures. Both sounds are analogous to tapping a drumhead that is pulled taut. Normally diastolic compliance is high and the chamber compliance declines if filling is increased. When end-diastolic pressures are elevated, the distensibility declines and one hears a low-pitch sound associated with filling.

3 Heart rate is likely to be increased as a compensation for reduced pump function due to the infarction. This is driven by sympathetic stimulation and vagal withdrawal.

4 Peripheral resistance is likely to be high even though arterial pressures are low. Remember that arterial pressure results from the interaction of the heart with the vascular system, and is not itself a reflection of arterial tone. In this case, reduced cardiac output would have resulted in a much lower arterial pressure had not the systemic arteries constricted. Preload volume is increased, as discussed in answer 1. If preload volume were increased and peripheral resistance increased in a normal heart, the arterial pressure would be very elevated. This can be illustrated using pressure–volume loops (see Chapter 13).

5 Systemic vascular resistance (SVR) = (mean arterial pressure (MAP) – right atrial pressure (RAP))/CO. From the data given, MAP is 82, RAP is 10, and CO is 3.0. Therefore, SVR = (82 – 10)/3 = 24. The units here are mmHg/L/min which are clinical units, but not those typically used to express resistance. The units that are more often used are dynes/s/cm^{-5}. To convert, you multiply 24 by 80 = 1920. Normal resistance is closer to 1200.

6 Net contractile function is reduced because of the recent heart injury (infarction). The heart with a heart attack is heterogeneous, with a very damaged region and remote compensating region that is closer to normal. The net effect, however, is still a decline in overall contractile function. Preload is elevated as noted, and afterload resistance increased. To improve cardiac output further and to reduce pulmonary oedema, you need to reduce preload with venodilators and diuretics, and lower afterload resistance with arterial vasodilators. Nitrates are an excellent class of drug for this purpose.

7 Cardiac output would very likely increase, and arterial pressures may not change much. If too much vasodilatation is induced, pressures will decline. However, with careful titration, one can often obtain an improvement in pump performance and coronary perfusion, and actually see a slight increase in pressure as the heart is better perfused.

8 Increasing contractile function is the last resort. One is particularly cautious in using inotropic therapy in a heart attack patient, because it is quite possible to make matters worse by increasing cardiac work and extending the territory of damage. Such patients often have coronary disease in places other than that directly responsible for the heart attack.

9 Myocardial flow occurs primarily during diastole, when myocardial pressure surrounding the arterioles is low and arterial perfusion pressure remains elevated (thanks to systemic vascular compliance and wave reflections). During systole, flow through the myocardium is inhibited by ventricular muscle contraction. So, if one had a method to enhance diastolic arterial pressures while simultaneously reducing systolic pressures, you are likely to improve cardiac perfusion while reducing ventricular load during ejection. Such a device exists and is called an **aortic counterpulsation balloon pump**. By inflating a balloon placed in the proximal descending aorta rapidly during diastole and deflating it during systole, you can augment the diastolic perfusion to the heart while improving forward output. In patients with ischaemic heart disease and reduced arterial pressures, this device is very useful indeed.

53 Case study: valvular heart disease

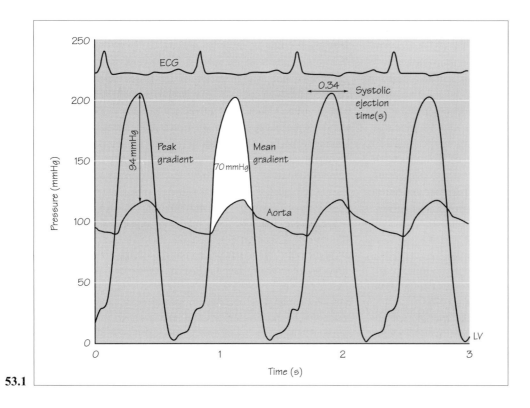

53.1

You are asked to supervise an exercise stress test on a 65-year-old man. He saw his doctor last week for exertional chest pain and mild dyspnoea. He has had chest discomfort for about a year, but the increased frequency of angina prompted him to see his doctor. He has chest pain when he walks more than one block, and if he continues he becomes breathless. He never has chest pain or dyspnoea at rest. He has no ankle swelling, orthopnoea, or paroxysmal nocturnal dyspnoea. When you examine him before the stress test, his blood pressure is 120/86, heart rate 82 and regular, jugular venous pressure 5 cmH$_2$O, and lungs are clear. His apex beat is slightly lateral to the midclavicular line and mildly sustained. He has a normal S$_1$ and a single S$_2$. An S$_4$ gallop is noted. He has a soft crescendo-decrescendo systolic murmur, best heard at the upper right sternal border, radiating to the carotids and the apex. The carotid pulses are delayed and diminished.

You call the referring doctor to discuss the signs and symptoms, cancel the stress test, and perform an echocardiogram instead.

Questions

1 What is the likely diagnosis based on the physical examination? What are the pathophysiological mechanisms underlying these findings?
2 He only had a soft systolic murmur. If you knew that his murmur last year was louder and harsher in intensity, would this have reassured you? What could go wrong if he did do the stress test?
3 What was likely to be observed on the echocardiogram and why?

Catheterization data: The patient is formally referred to you, and you recommend valve replacement. He undergoes cardiac catheterization, and the haemodynamic data are shown in Fig. 53.1. Cardiac output is 5.2 L/min, and heart rate is 77. There is no significant coronary artery disease.

4 The aortic valve area can be estimated by the simplified formula:

Valve area = cardiac output/√pressure gradient

Based on the data given, what is his estimated valve area?
5 When admitted for surgery, he complains of chest pain. The intern orders sublingual nitroglycerin for him. Why is this a bad idea? What is the chest pain due to? What therapeutic options are available for protracted chest pain in this case?

Answers

1 He is likely to have severe aortic stenosis. The crescendo-decrescendo systolic murmur usually arises from stenosis of either the aortic or pulmonary valve. The stenotic valve creates turbulence during ejection that causes a murmur. The murmur gets louder as flow increases during ejection, then diminishes as flow decreases. This murmur is transmitted to the carotid arteries because of the high velocity of the ejected blood. The apical murmur is probably caused by high-frequency vibration of the aortic valve during ejection and can sometimes be louder than that at the sternal border.

Aortic stenosis causes left ventricular hypertrophy, which displaces the apex beat laterally. The apex beat can be sustained because the ventricle takes longer to empty. The carotid pulse contour reflects flow across the aortic valve. Because peak ejection flow is delayed and decreased in aortic stenosis, the carotid pulses are delayed and diminished.

2 The loudness of murmur depends on *flow* across the valve; therefore it may not reflect the severity of valve stenosis. In the case of aortic stenosis, other physical examination parameters are more indicative of the severity of valve stenosis. As valve area becomes smaller, the peak loudness of the murmur occurs later in systole. This is presumably due to the difficulty in opening the valve. In severe aortic stenosis left ventricular stroke volume is decreased. This manifests as low-amplitude carotid pulsation with a delayed peak (***pulsus parvus et tardus***).

Normally, the aortic valve closes before the pulmonary valve, causing splitting of S_2. During inspiration more blood volume is returned to the right heart and the pulmonary valve closes even later. The increased splitting of S_2 during inspiration is termed physiological splitting. In severe aortic stenosis, the ejection time becomes longer, and the aortic valve closes later. This may eliminate splitting of S_2 (single S_2), or create paradoxical splitting.

If this murmur was previously louder, it would suggest that flow across the valve has decreased as the stenosis worsened. Decrease in flow (lower cardiac output) is an ominous sign of a failing left ventricle or a decrease in valve size. This is not reassuring.

During exercise, blood vessels dilate and peripheral resistance decreases. When the peripheral resistance falls, the blood pressure tends to fall. Normal individuals compensate by increasing stroke volume and heart rate. However, this patient cannot increase his stroke volume because of the tight aortic valve. When blood pressure falls, coronary perfusion decreases, and the subendocardial area of the hypertrophied ventricle is not perfused adequately. As heart rate and oxygen demand increase, the supply and demand mismatch may worsen and cause ischaemia. If a significant portion of the myocardium is affected, cardiac output can fall, causing a further drop in coronary perfusion and further worsening ischaemia. This vicious cycle can continue until the patient drops dead, an event that may not look particularly good on your record.

3 The echocardiogram showed uniform left ventricular hypertrophy. His left ventricular ejection fraction was estimated at 45%, and the aortic valve appeared calcified with impaired cusp mobility. Doppler studies showed the peak instantaneous gradient across the aortic valve was 98 mmHg with a mean gradient of 68 mmHg. Estimated aortic valve area was 0.6 cm².

The most common cause of aortic stenosis in this age group is calcific degeneration of the aortic cusps. The valvular pathology leads to left ventricular hypertrophy, a pressure gradient, and impaired emptying of the chamber, which were all demonstrated on the echocardiogram.

4 Using the formula the estimated valve area is 0.62 cm². This formula is a simplified version of the Gorlin formula, which states that the valve area is related to cardiac output, and inversely related to mean pressure gradient, systolic ejection period, and the gravitational acceleration constant. In most cases, the systolic ejection period multiplied by the acceleration constant is close to 1, so that term is not used in the estimate formula.

5 This patient's left ventricle (LV) needs all the help it can get to eject an adequate supply of blood through the pin-hole-sized aortic valve. Nitroglycerin is primarily a venodilator, and it will pool his blood in the veins. This will reduce blood returning to the heart and decrease preload. Even though the ejection fraction is only 45%, his thick LV still has high contractility and a steep end-systolic pressure–volume relation. This means that he is very sensitive to preload changes, and a slight drop in preload volume can drop blood pressure significantly, which will decrease coronary perfusion, worsen subendocardial ischaemia, decrease systolic dysfunction, lower blood pressure, and so on. Thus, nitrates are a bad idea. β-adrenergic blockers or calcium-channel blockers are also not good because they can reduce contractility. Calcium-channel blockers can also dilate peripheral arterioles and reduce blood pressure further.

What *can* you do? You may actually give some fluid to increase preload and increase cardiac output. The other mode of therapy, if the valve cannot be replaced promptly, is intra-aortic balloon counter-pulsation. This can improve coronary perfusion in some cases and relieve subendocardial ischaemia.

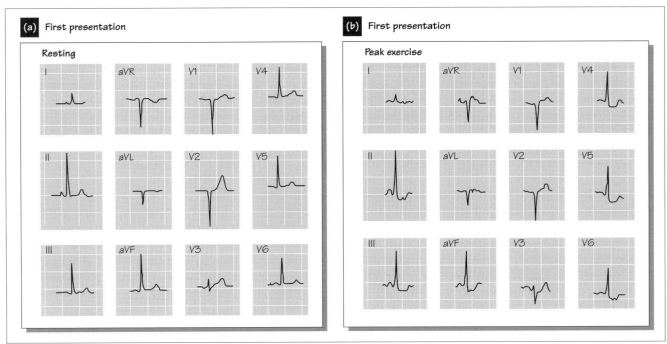

(a) First presentation — Resting — I, aVR, V1, V4, II, aVL, V2, V5, III, aVF, V3, V6

(b) First presentation — Peak exercise — I, aVR, V1, V4, II, aVL, V2, V5, III, aVF, V3, V6

54.1

A 53-year-old woman presents with a prolonged episode of chest discomfort. The discomfort is under her sternum, and is a squeezing feeling that extends to her left arm and jaws. She has had this on and off for 3 months. It usually occurs when she goes up two flights of stairs, but never when resting. Tonight, the discomfort began while walking to buy cigarettes, and lasted for 40 min. She has no known medical problems and has not seen a doctor in more than 20 years. Her last menstrual period was 4 years ago. She takes no medications. Her family history is only significant in that her father died of a heart attack when he was 74 years old.

On examination, she appears well and in no acute distress. Her height is 5 feet 6 inches (1.68 m) and weight 120 pounds (55 kg). Her blood pressure is 132/84 and heart rate 74. There is no jugular venous distension, and her lungs are clear to percussion and auscultation. Cardiac examination is normal. Her abdomen is benign, and there is no oedema. Pulses are full and equal bilaterally without thrills. An ECG shows normal sinus rhythm without abnormalities.

Questions

1 Is this angina pectoris?
2 What predisposing factors does she have for coronary artery disease (CAD)? What other risk factors might she have? Could this have been a myocardial infarction (MI)?

She is admitted for monitoring. Serial serum enzyme tests are negative, and ECG remains normal after 18 h. Fasting serum

glucose is 92, and fasting lipid profile is: total cholesterol 198, HDL 36, LDL 137, and triglycerides 126. She undergoes a graded exercise test for 12 min, and has chest discomfort with the ECG abnormalities shown in Fig. 54.1(b). Her blood pressure rose from 124/78 to 180/76 at peak exercise. Her heart rate rose from 78 to 143. The chest discomfort resolved within 5 min of stopping exercise, and the ECG returned to normal. Coronary angiography showed a focal 70% narrowing in the right coronary artery and a focal 30% narrowing in the left anterior descending artery (LAD). She is treated with anti-ischaemic medicines, advised on low-cholesterol diets and aerobic exercise, instructed on the use of sublingual nitroglycerin, started on aspirin and atenolol, and discharged. She agrees to stop smoking. She will return for follow-up in 7 days for another exercise test.

3 What serum enzymes are useful in diagnosing myocardial damage?
4 Why not perform angioplasty on the coronary lesions?
5 Her cholesterol is not high. Why a low-cholesterol diet? Would lowering blood cholesterol help her existing CAD? What other risk factors can she modify?
6 Why perform a follow-up exercise test?

Second presentation: The patient does well on the medicines and stops smoking. She has no chest discomfort even during vigorous exercise. However, within the week she is awakened from sleep by the same chest discomfort. As nitroglycerin is

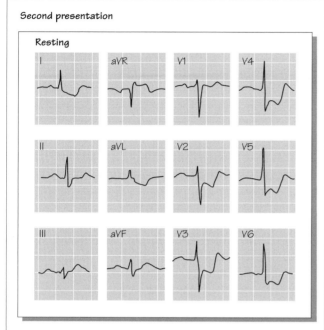

Second presentation

Resting

I aVR V1 V4

II aVL V2 V5

III aVF V3 V6

54.2

ineffective, she is brought to hospital. Her ECG is shown in Fig. 54.2. She is given oxygen, aspirin, intravenous nitroglycerin and heparin, and her chest discomfort then recedes. It lasted for 35 min. Because of recurrent chest discomfort in hospital, she has another coronary angiogram. This shows the same 70% narrowing in the right coronary artery, but the 30% LAD narrowing has now grown to 99%. Cardiac enzymes are still negative.

7 What does the new ECG show? What is your diagnosis? How is the pathophysiology of the current chest discomfort different from her previous effort-related angina?
8 Do the ECG abnormalities correlate with the coronary angiogram? What is the 'culprit' lesion? How could the LAD lesion progress so fast? Why use aspirin and heparin? How about thrombolytic agents?

Answers

1 This sounds like angina. The location, radiation and type of discomfort are consistent with cardiac ischaemic pain.
2 Her risk factors for CAD are smoking and being postmenopausal. Her family history is *not* positive for premature CAD, because her father was 74 when he had his MI. She does not have hypertension. We do not yet know her cholesterol levels, or whether she is diabetic.

The traditional dividing line between 'angina' and possible MI is 30 min of discomfort. Because her discomfort lasted more than 30 min, it is possible she suffered an MI, even with

a normal ECG. To determine whether a MI occurred, look for evidence of myocardial damage such as cardiac-specific serum enzymes.
3 The most commonly used enzyme is creatine kinase. A rise in serum levels of the cardiac specific (MB) isoform is seen with myocardial damage. Cardiac troponins are useful in confirming myocardial damage.
4 She does not have unstable angina at this point, and her effort tolerance is reasonable. Such patients have a good prognosis whether they take medicines or have single-vessel angioplasty. A recent study showed that angioplasty was no better than medicines for single-vessel CAD.
5 Her cholesterol was not high, but recent studies indicate that lowering LDL cholesterol below ~110 mg/dl may stabilize coronary lesions and possibly cause regression of CAD. However, greater effects were seen on reduced incidence of unstable angina or MI. These may be due to reducing the lipid-rich area of plaques and making them less susceptible to rupture.

The most important thing was to stop smoking. Reducing cholesterol is a secondary prevention. Another risk factor is lack of oestrogen. Postmenopausal women with CAD may benefit from hormone replacement therapy.
6 Reasons for exercise testing are: diagnosis; prognosis; and to test effectiveness of treatment. Here, we want to know if her anti-anginal regimen is adequate.
7 The ECG shows marked ST segment depression in the precordial (V1–V6) and lateral (I and aVL) leads. She has cardiac ischaemia, either due to unstable angina or a MI. The chest discomfort occurred during sleep, so it is unstable angina. She could additionally have an MI, as ST segment elevation is not always present in MI.

Cardiac ischaemia occurs when myocardial oxygen demand exceeds supply. This typically happens with exertion in CAD patients, because bloodflow through the stenosis is usually adequate during rest. Rest ischaemia is caused when the oxygen supply falls below that required for even basal myocardial metabolic needs. This implies a more occlusive lesion, such as unstable angina. It is believed that unstable angina is initiated by plaque rupture, causing aggregation of platelets and fibrin deposition. This can not only cause stenosis, but also vasospasm.
8 The angiogram suggests the 'culprit' is the LAD lesion. It is tighter, and stenotic enough to cause rest angina. The ECG abnormalities are consistent with the ischaemic area being that served by the LAD. Unstable angina involves platelets and the clotting cascade. Thus it makes sense to use inhibitors of platelet aggregation (aspirin) and anticoagulants (heparin). Clot formation and dissolution are dynamic processes, and although aspirin and heparin cannot directly disperse clots, they can promote resolution. Thrombolytics make theoretical sense, but in trials no improvement in outcome of unstable angina patients was seen, and morbidity was *higher*.

55 Case studies: arrhythmias

Case 1

Initial presentation: A 64-year-old man with a history of long-standing hypertension and diabetes presents complaining of shortness of breath and weakness. He has orthopnoea but no chest pain. His physical examination is notable for a heart rate of 150 beats/min, a blood pressure of 100/70, and a respiratory rate of 24. There are bilateral crackles a third of the way up the lung fields, the first heart sound is soft, and there is a summation gallop. His ECG is shown in Fig. 55.1(a). Carotid sinus massage then changes the rhythm to the one shown in Fig. 55.1(b).

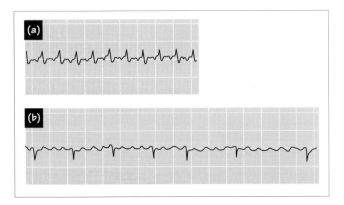

Figure 55.1 (a) Lead II. Atrial flutter with 2 : 1 conduction. Heart rate 150 beats/min. (b) Lead II. Arial flutter after carotid sinus massage. Note the characteristic sawtooth pattern of flutter waves, and AV conduction of 4 : 1 to 6 : 1.

Questions

1 What is the ventricular rate in Fig. 55.1(a)? Is this a ventricular or supraventricular arrhythmia?
2 Based on the effect of carotid sinus massage, what is the diagnosis? How does carotid sinus massage affect the ventricular response?
3 What pharmacological agents can be used to slow the ventricular response?

Results of treatment: The patient is admitted to hospital and begun on digitalis and amiodarone. The next morning he feels better, but his pulse is irregularly irregular with an apical pulse of 110 and a radial pulse of 70. An ECG is shown in Fig. 55.2.

4 What is the rhythm now? Is the change from the day before common?
5 Is the current antiarrhythmic regimen appropriate?
6 What other therapy may be indicated? Why?

Answers

1 The ventricular rate is 150 beats/min. The narrow QRS complex implies that the tachycardia involves the atrioventricular

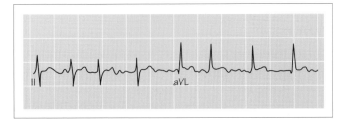

Figure 55.2 Leads II and aVL. Atrial flutter has degenerated into atrial fibrillation. Note the irregularity of the ventricular rate, indicated by the varying intervals between the QRS complexes.

node (AVN), and is therefore supraventricular. The differential diagnosis for this tachycardia includes AV nodal re-entrant tachycardia, atrial flutter, or sinus tachycardia. Atrial fibrillation is unlikely because the rhythm is regular.

2 Carotid sinus massage demonstrates the sawtooth pattern of flutter waves, particularly in the inferior leads (II, III, aVF). This proves that the initial rhythm was atrial flutter with 2 : 1 conduction (i.e. only one of every two atrial waves is conducted through the AVN to the ventricle). Because the flutter waves have a rate of nearly 300 beats/min, the ventricular rate is 150 beats/min. Carotid sinus massage increases vagal tone, slowing conduction through the AVN and increasing AV block.

3 β-blockers, digoxin, Ca^{2+}-channel blockers and adenosine slow conduction through the AVN. This slows the ventricular rate, allowing adequate time for left ventricular filling, and relieving the symptoms of left heart failure (shortness of breath, weakness, orthopnoea).

4 This is atrial fibrillation; note the irregularly irregular ventricular rate. Atrial flutter is an unstable rhythm, and commonly degenerates into atrial fibrillation.

5 Yes. Amiodarone and digoxin are commonly used to treat atrial arrhythmias. Digoxin helps to slow the ventricular rate by increasing vagal tone at the AVN. Amiodarone similarly helps to slow the ventricular response. Amiodarone is also used to cardiovert patients with atrial arrhythmias back into sinus rhythm and/or help maintain sinus rhythm once they have been electrically cardioverted.

6 Patients with intermittent or persistent atrial fibrillation should receive anticoagulation because of the risk of embolic stroke. In this patient, who seems to be having his first episode of atrial fibrillation, electrical cardioversion should be attempted if amiodarone does not convert the rhythm to sinus.

Case 2

Initial presentation: A 55-year-old man presents with a 24-h history of shortness of breath and palpitations. He has mild dizziness and diaphoresis. There is no prior record of MI, but he has longstanding hypertension and cigarette smoking. His blood pressure is 80/52, heart rate is 186 beats/min and regular, and his respiratory rate is 26. There are crackles bilaterally, jugular venous pressure (JVP) is raised, and a III/VI holosystolic murmur at the apex radiates to the axilla but not the neck. His ECG is shown in Fig. 55.3.

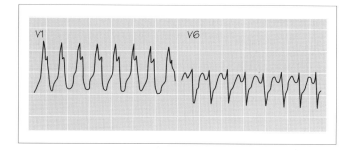

Figure 55.3 Leads V1 and V6. Ventricular tachycardia. Heart rate 186 beats/min. The QRS complex is abnormally wide. There is a large primary R wave in lead V1, and exaggerated R wave, leading to an R/S ratio < 1, in V6.

Questions

1 What does the III/VI holosystolic murmur indicate?
2 Is this tachycardia more likely supraventricular or ventricular? Why? What is the axis and the QRS morphology?
3 Why is he short of breath and hypotensive? Why is his JVP elevated?
4 What would be appropriate treatment?

Results of treatment: The patient receives lidocaine. This fails to convert him to sinus rhythm and he is therefore electrically cardioverted. The resulting ECG is shown in Fig. 55.4.

5 What is the rhythm now?
6 What is the likely cause of his acute presentation?
7 What would be the appropriate evaluation with this information?

Answers

1 This indicates a moderate murmur of mitral regurgitation (see Chapter 49).
2 This rhythm is most likely ventricular in origin. When a patient has a wide-complex tachycardia, the differential diagnosis is ventricular tachycardia (VT) vs supraventricular tachycardia with aberrant conduction (i.e. the tachycardia is conducted with a bundle branch block). A wide variety of clinical and ECG criteria aid in distinguishing between these possibilities. The most important clinical criterion is whether the patient has a history of heart disease (see below). If this is the case, and in particular if there is a history of MI, the most likely origin of the tachycardia is ventricular, because an infarct creates a substrate for re-entry. ECG criteria which suggest a ventricular origin include: (i) a very wide QRS complex; (ii) an extreme axis; (iii) evidence of atrial-ventricular dissociation; (iv) certain specific QRS morphologies. This patient's QRS morphology is that of a right bundle.

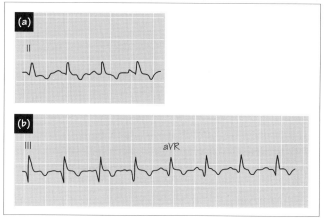

Figure 55.4 Leads II, III, aVR. After cardioversion, patient restored to sinus rhythm. Heart rate 95 beats/min. Note the exaggerated Q waves and elevation of the ST segment, indicating an old inferior wall MI.

Note the terminal S waves in V6, and the R in V1. The extreme axis, the very wide QRS duration and the morphology (R/S < 1 in V6 and the large primary R in V1) suggest the rhythm is VT.
3 He is short of breath and hypotensive because the tachycardia does not allow enough time for ventricular filling. Therefore cardiac output is low, causing hypotension, and left atrial pressure is high. The high left atrial pressure has backed up into his pulmonary capillaries, causing pulmonary oedema and breathlessness. His increased JVP is caused by raised central venous pressure, indicative of inadequate right ventricular function. His arrhythmia is therefore causing congestive heart failure.
4 Treatment requires cardioversion to sinus rhythm with either appropriate drugs (lidocaine, procainamide, or amiodarone) or electrical cardioversion. Because this patient's symptoms indicate that his arrhythmia is causing his heart to fail, immediate conversion to sinus rhythm is mandatory. Therefore in this case electrical cardioversion is preferable.
5 The rhythm is now sinus, with the rate of 95 beats/min.
6 He has evidence on his ECG of an inferior wall MI (note the Q waves in leads II, III, aVF with slight ST elevation). The aetiology of his ventricular tachycardia is likely to be re-entry into left ventricular (LV) scar caused by an undetected recent acute MI.
7 Following stabilization, appropriate treatment includes evaluation of LV function and of coronary anatomy.

In this case, the patient had severe inoperable coronary artery disease and poor LV function. Because poor ejection fraction identifies high risk for recurrent VT and sudden death, the patient underwent electrophysiology testing and was readily inducible into hypotensive VT. This indicated: (i) that he was at a high risk to spontaneously develop VT again; (ii) that his tachycardia was fast enough to lower his cardiac output dangerously. His already poor LV function meant that he would not be able to tolerate tachycardia. He therefore subsequently underwent successful placement of an internal cardioverter-defibrillator and has since been stable.

Index